T0374314

Logical H.I.T.

Logical H.I.T.

A Means To Fight For Your Greatest Value: Your Happiness, Your Life

By Alexander Fee

iUniverse, Inc.

New York   Bloomington

Logical H.I.T.
A Means To Fight For Your Greatest
Value: Your Happiness, Your Life

*You should not undertake any diet/exercise regimen recommended
in this book before consulting your personal physician. Neither the
author nor the publisher shall be responsible or liable for any loss or
damage allegedly arising as a consequence of your use or application
of any information or suggestions contained in this book.*

iUniverse books may be ordered through booksellers or by contacting:

iUniverse
1663 Liberty Drive
Bloomington, IN 47403
www.iuniverse.com
1-800-Authors (1-800-288-4677)

ISBN: 978-1-4401-3653-5 (pbk)
ISBN: 978-1-4401-3652-8 (ebk)

Printed in the United States of America

iUniverse rev. date: 6/24/2009

This book is dedicated to the individuals out there who still hold onto their dream in the face of adversity, denouncers, and critics…whatever that dream may be. To those who stand in inexorable defiance of the lesser than what they are capable of achieving. To those who stand with fervescent passion and in loving defense for the capabilities of man's mind and all of his potentialities. To those who stare into the world, not with anxiety and fear, but with elated anticipation of what they can be, of what they can create! To those who are the smallest minority—the individual and their means of individuality… this book is dedicated to Man's Mind.

In memory of all the individuals of history that moved us forward, but seldom, if ever, are given the respect that they rightly deserve...individuals who are now in the process of being lost to the abyss of ignorance's obscurity. But we must never forget! I write this book in memory of Mike Mentzer, Ayn Rand, Arthur Jones, Isaac Newton, Galileo Galilei, Aristotle, Nikola Tesla and others of history's past that gave us fire to light our world and the wheel that opened it to be ours to take, but all who have already succumb to that void of anonymity.

Acknowledgements

_"If I have seen further than others, it is by
standing upon the shoulders of giants."_
Sir Isaac Newton

I would like to show my appreciation towards the groundbreaking works of the late Arthur Jones, founder of Nautilus Sports/Medical Industries and MedX Corporation, for establishing the theory of High Intensity Training, for being one of the first (and one of the very few) individuals to bring rationality and logic to a field that is exceedingly misunderstood and far too underappreciated, and for being one of the last truly free men in this dying world of mediocrity and sacrifice.

John Little deserves my greatest gratitude for taking the time to teach a young fool how to open his eyes. John Little is the innovator of Max Contraction™ and co-innovator of Power Factor Training ™ and Static Contraction Training™, a columnist in Ironman magazine as well as the coauthor, along with Dr. Doug McGuff, of the most important book on exercise today (Body by Science), but more than that, John has been one of very few individuals in my life to have a hand in the development of my intellect for the better. So all that

I would like to say is, thank you John for being one of today's few truly good and great men.

However, where John Little was my spark, Mike Mentzer was my fuel. Mike Mentzer, world-renowned Objectivist bodybuilder/philosopher, writer and creator of Heavy Duty™ training, has been the model for my intellectual and physical growth. Mentzer epitomized the Greek ideal of "A healthy mind in a health body" and showed thousands of young and old bodybuilders that you can live life, achieving both the practical and the ideal. And although his passing closed a chapter in bodybuilding's chronicle of heroic physiques, his personality and magnanimous intellect remain strong and true.

Ayn Rand, the architect of the Objectivist philosophy and author of the world-renown novels The Fountainhead, Atlas Shrugged, We the Living and Anthem, is one of the first and few individuals that stood tall against today's rampaging storm of compromise, self-sacrifice and irrationality—holding that it is man's right to live for his own sake, that life without sacrifice and compromise is not only alright, but just! Her ideas have stimulated the minds of countless individuals…individuals thirsty for more than what the majority, the church and the government say is adequate for an individual. Dr. Leonard Peikoff, PhD, Ayn Rand's intellectual heir and the world's foremost authority on Ayn Rand's philosophy, with his tireless integrity and sense of justice, has made it his life's work to spread the philosophy of Objectivism and to nourish America's dwindling flame of reason and logic in the effort of bring mankind out of this rapid fall towards, not a new dark age, but a darker age, one devoid of ideology and reason. Ayn Rand and Dr. Leonard Peikoff, it would require numerous pages to express my gratitude for their efforts, but all that I would like to say is, thank you for fighting for your ideals and for never compromising on your principles.

I would also like to express the deepest gratitude for my dear friend Koko Kitae for her beautiful cover that arouses the deepest paroxysm of joy. The participants of the Haircut Study who inspired the instigation of this book, I would like to thank all of them for their help in proving and revealing truths of the human body for my book and my career. And I would to thank my good friend Brandon Robataille for his aid in the refining of many of the practical aspects of the book.

Contents

Introduction

The title of this book might be somewhat confusing and may require a little more of an explanation for a number of individuals. The title H.I.T. is an acronym condensing a scientific theory of bodybuilding exercise: High Intensity Training. I would like to state at this moment in time, so no misconceptions are drawn, that this method of bodybuilding exercise was not created by me. It was theoretically ensconced almost forty years ago by the late Arthur Jones, and was fundamentally completed by the late Mike Mentzer approximately 12 years ago. The practical application of this "type" of training (i.e. hard work), no matter how crude it was in its application, has been used for thousands of years. Have you ever heard the story of Milo of Croton, the legend of an Olympian who carried a calf everyday for four years and grew progressively stronger as the calf grew progressively larger, or seen pictures of the Farnese Hercules that displays the perfect anatomical proportions for an individual of truly great muscularity that would be IMPOSSIBLE to sculpt without an actual model who possessed those exact proportions?

The significance of my use of the term "Logical" in the title is to signify that this book is a logical view of the theory of high intensity training, thus this book emboldens Mike Mentzer's, *Heavy Duty*™ philosophy of bodybuilding exercise and the Objectivist philosophy of life. (I would like to state here that I am an Objectivist, a student of Ayn Rand's philosophy. However, I am neither an expert nor an authority on Ayn Rand's philosophy of Objectivism, and I do not represent the Ayn Rand Institute.)

The issue of separating my work from the popular orthodoxy of high intensity training is for the reason that proper high intensity training has unfortunately been misconstrued by many of its activists. The history of the H.I.T. methodology is highlighted with contrasting images of the legendary workouts of Casey Viator instructed by the late Arthur Jones to the colossal, teratological workouts of six-time Mr. Olympia Dorian Yates performed in an outright dangerous explosive style, not unlike that of an Olympic weightlifter. All of which today is now being supplemented with the image of the newly emerging HIT facilities that advocate a clutter of contradictory misinformation and perpetuate ignorance into the only rational method of bodybuilding exercise.

This book however is not a compilation of the history of high intensity training, advocating the contradictory information still held onto by the traditionalists of the theory, doing so with the hope of the possibility that if I present enough of a variety of routines that one routine, out of an extensive list, "might" work for you. No, this book *is* an elucidation of proper logical bodybuilding exercise that is conducted in the most efficacious manner possible and performed in the absolute least amount time required to stimulate the desired results, allowing you to reach your full muscular potential in the shortest time possible.

This book makes use of an extensive philosophic-scientific context within which to present my knowledge of high intensity "global metabolic conditioning" body-building stress physiology. The philosophic content this book deals with is fundamental, yet still comprehensive, allowing you to achieve a fundamental understanding of all the sciences.

So, if you are weary of endless hours of working out in the gym with little in the way of manifesting results… if you are morally shaken and intellectually uncertain of truth and of your self-worth, I implore you to study this book with an inquisitive mind. To actively question everything you do not understand and to make an effort to understand the truth in this book by means of your faculty of reason. Some individuals will find some of the terminology a bit daunting or see it as "too intellectual" for them, but do not become disheartened. Merely write down the words you do not understand and look them up, you might even make the delightful discovery that they prove of great value in your future thinking and learning. However, understand as well that achieving an extraordinarily well developed physique cannot be fully appreciated nor even attained unless your mind develops to meet the demand of such a task.

The content in the first six chapters of this book deals with is theoretical, while after that I will be presenting the practical, "how to do it" information that will instruct you on how to train in the most efficacious manner possible. But you can't just skip to that point straight away without grasping the theory itself. This book is not meant to merely give you a training routine and expect you to blindly follow it…of what benefit would you gain from that, save for a routine that works despite your understanding—but will usually not yield any results unless you are dispelled of the blinding myths and misconceptions that will almost certainly restrict you until you come to grasp the absolute *necessity* of why you *must* train in such a manner. This book is intended to reveal to you a universally valid theory of bodybuilding exercise and the method of acquiring *intellectual certainty*; moreover, to entice you to think for yourself and to question the unsubstantiated traditions and the accepted edicts of the majority consensus.

No, you should not be concerned with developing an open mind—deeming every concept as having some validity—while reading the information in this book, but an active mind. One that deals with ideas seriously, devoted to separate truth from falsehood. Spend the time necessary to understand and grasp the logic of my ideas and take the time to reflect upon the premises and concepts presented in this work. If at first you do not understand some of the philosophic concepts in this book, sit down with a dictionary and reread and re-reread this book until you are able to grasp the meaning and importance of these concepts in one's conceptual context. This book is meant to assist you in selfishly and intelligently taking control of *your* body and *your* life.

"I think it is most important to discover as quickly as possible in your physical culture career not how much exercise is necessary, but how little!"

Harry Paschall

1

All That Glitters is not Gold

"Truth, like gold, is to be obtained not by its growth, but by washing away from it all that is not gold."

Leo Nikolaevich Tolstoy

Today man's mind is under attack, but not by whom you would imagine...nor wish to covet in nightmare. The results of the efforts of these intellectual assailants is that today there is a total systemic deterioration of man's certainty concerning his values, his morals, his knowledge and even his existence! Those who attack and aim to render the mind of man impotent are today's admired intellectuals.

These antagonists of reason convene in a second-handed Ivory Tower and comedown merely to fill the minds of the helplessly confused and innocently un-knowing individuals with arbitrary mystical philosophies and pragmatic ultimatums. Their intellectual vomit stating that there is no certainty and that reality is purely subjective. They declare that nothing is the same for any two individuals; that everyone is different, based on the premise that an objective reality does not really exist. And when these intellectuals are confronted with reason and objective evidence they scoff at those who believe that

1

man is able to find valid truth—they protract from argument, threatened by the inescapable requisite of using reason to prove a point.

The realm of bodybuilding is but merely one example of today's intellectual erosion and moral deprivation… epitomizing an oasis of fool's gold. When entering into any endeavor in life, including that of bodybuilding, with an "open-mind" all bets are off and the weltering blitz commences. And the first and foremost barrage digs in deep and is the cause for the dramatic decrease in the interest in bodybuilding today: irrationalism, the obfuscation of certainty in absolutes and its corollary: the desolation of one's self-esteem (their self-appraisal of their worthiness of self-improvement).

The detriment of such irrational philosophical premises begins with the neophytic bodybuilder's first tie to those who become his physique idols: the goal of actualizing the glory of one's muscular potential, of being a physical testament to one's own efficacy as a human being. As the result of this self-declaration of worth, they setoff for the one source of information that the culture tells them is the only source of bodybuilding information and to unquestionably obey it if one so desires results: the muscle magazines, i.e., the advice of the profession's experts.

Thus, after riffling through the pages of a few muscle magazines, choosing a routine that was used by an individual that possesses the kind of physique they desire—ignorant of genetically predisposed individual physical potential—, they stick to that routine, faithfully, for a few months or so. However, after a month or so of mediocre growth, followed by a period of muscular stagnation, even retrogression, they find themselves in a state of confusion, and even worse, after a period of deliberation and restudy among their accumulating collection of muscle magazines they begin to panic when they can't find an answer as to why. They are unable to find a straight answer out of the cumulative inventory of repetitive articles, all saying the same damn thing of "everybody is different and you have to find what works for you."

Panic stricken, with no solid grounds to even start their search for the answers they desire, they launch with reckless abandon into consuming expensive "muscle building" concoctions that promise to be the philosopher's stone of muscle growth in addition to flying through magazines, books, websites and fellow bodybuilders in the gym…all for even the slightest trace of productive advice. Their sources answer with, "Try this or that supplement, it worked for this or that pro" or, "Try this or that routine, because everyone is different and you have to find what works for you"…for all intents and purposes they acquire all that today's era of bodybuilding has to offer—blank out.

The hallmark of today's bodybuilder is quite literally a state of almost perpetual confusion, as almost all bodybuilders today fail to achieve their goals rather than succeed. The undertone of this chapter, not surprisingly, seems to resound as the question, is bodybuilding even worth doing? …But just for a moment, close your eyes and imagine yourself with a tremendously striking physique. A physique highlighted with deeply carved abs, chiseled and powerful pecs, strong muscular arms that command attention from everyone, shoulders that cannot be concealed by even a burlap sack, a back that ripples with detail and Herculean muscularity, all finished off with legs that could bear the weight of the world.

It becomes quite clear why so many individuals find bodybuilding so attractive and worth pursuing. However, upon embarking upon their noble quest of self-improvement, bodybuilders immediately arrive at a crossroad that leads to other crossroads that carry on until the inconclusive intellectual welter brings them right back to where they started.

They return with a few elements that seem to be consistent in this mass of contradictory bodybuilding information; most of all there is a consistency of there being a need to lift weights. However, the topic of weight lifting is a subject that most people become one-sided on without, for the most part, rational justification.

One activist will protest the idea of weight lifting as just being dangerous; concurring that the body is bearing strain under a heavy load, but implying that it is the precursor of inevitable physical injury. Or believing that with heavy weight lifting one will develop uncontrollably and unceasingly until they reach the incredible muscular levels of today's heavily muscled professional bodybuilders. As a result, they employ very light weights, high repetitions and avoid any real effort.

While others opposing this view will argue the subject—fighting to the death—that, with a mindless and religious devotion, weight lifting is the greatest thing one can do for themselves; condemning those whom do not partake with a sneer and a cold shoulder. They crow that unbounded exercise will enable you to live longer with a stronger heart—mainly due to the orthodoxy of cardiovascular exercise—and that ballistic weight "throwing" (as few individuals utilizing exercise equipment actually muscularly *lift* weights) will bestow upon your body gargantuan muscles and youthful vitality.

However, these two tribes of disillusion are forging all of their premises on traditional stigmas and arbitrary notions that lack any signs of rational foundation. Later on in this book, I will be laying down the truth of the matter and showing you both the positive and negative potential properties of exercise, using scientific, objective facts of human physiology and basic physics.

I will entice you further by stating a blunt—and should be—obvious fact, that aerobic activity (i.e. running, swimming, biking and so on) and conventional weight lifting exercise for health benefits are almost utterly worthless, as we will see later on. Due to their long duration and lack of a productive physiologic stimulus, these forms of physical activities provide no physiologic benefit, but they can, and usually do, wear down the body and can quickly lead to overtraining—which is quite the precarious problem, indeed.

The major philosophic thesis of this book is that, if you do not have a firm intellectual grasp and guidance by a valid theory, in any aspect and issue in life, you cannot possibly be certain that you are proceeding in the right direction. If you were confronted with a torrent of intersecting roads and twisting highways between you and the destination you desire to reach that is hundreds of miles away, would you set off with not even the slightest clue of how to get there? Even as an only a semi-rational individual you would not, as you would wander about, soon becoming lost and eventually lose all interest in your goal of reaching your desired destination.

In order to get from your current location to your sought after destination you would consult a *map*—a map being a *theory* of a specific aspect of reality and a guide for successful human action. Ideally, you would consult a particular and equally productive theory for successful human action in bodybuilding with the intention of increasing muscular size and strength...and such a theory does exist. Furthermore, just as there *is* and can *only* be one correct immutable theory for a map, there *is* and can *only* be one correct theory of bodybuilding exercise...if two maps showed two completely different locations for one particular city they could not both be correct.

The correct theory of bodybuilding exercise must provide the apex of possible physiological benefits in addition to being the most economically efficient with results regarding the time required to obtain them. The only <u>correct</u> form of exercise one can perform with the intention of an increase of muscle size and strength is high intensity training, due to the objective facts of reality that make this theory valid. Now, do not start lecturing me on how big some professional bodybuilder's arms are, while pointing to such muscle mass as proof of his great knowledge on the subject of exercise and the legitimacy of his method. The production of any given result (no matter how spectacular it may be) proves nothing beyond the simple fact that a particular method has the potential of producing a given result, eventually, within specific conditions. In the case of almost all of the professional bodybuilders today, most do not even have the slightest clue of why or how they were able to attain their stature. I can tell you without a doubt that it was not specifically due to their training, but their almost superhuman genetics and their frightening consumption of growth promoting drugs that allow them to progress *in spite of* their counterproductive efforts in the gym.

All such individuals *would* have attained greater or, at the very least, their current muscular mass faster, requiring almost inestimably lesser time spent in the gym with the implementation of a high intensity training program.

*   *   *

It is only with a valid theory that progress in the desired direction will be immediate, significant and uninterrupted. A valid theory will be the one and only method capable of reaching an ultimate goal or standard, whether it is actualizing your full muscular potential in as little as years time (high intensity training) or raising the standard of life of and wealth of man (laissez-faire capitalism) or a philosophy for living on earth as a prosperous human being, not shackled by a morality that damns him for existing (Objectivism). The application of a valid theory results in almost unimaginable progress, so much so that most people who refuse that there is only one valid theory of any aspect of reality attack it with vicious and deceitful spite, attempting to silence it by force of consensus or political pull.

Part I

Rational by Choice—Man by Choice

"Voting for politicians that tell you what you want to hear has all but destroyed civilization—giving in to outrage in the hope of avoiding trouble has all but destroyed freedom—and looking for the easy road to success in bodybuilding has all but destroyed the actually great potential value of weight training. Which perpetuates the politicians, pleases the perpetrators of outrages and pads the pocket of a pack of predators in the field of bodybuilding."

Arthur Jones

"Education rears disciples, imitators, and routinists, not pioneers of new ideas and creative geniuses. The schools are not nurseries of progress and improvement, but conservatories of tradition and unvarying modes of thought."

Ludwig Von Mises, economist and philosopher

2

Why Bodybuilders Need a Rational Philosophy

"Nature, to be apprehended, must be obeyed."

Ayn Rand

Acknowledging that the information in this book represents a clear-cut certainty of universally valid truths, the skeptics and mystics among the experts today (whether we are dealing with exercise physiologists, physicists or philosophers) question how I can possibly prove, or dismiss the notion that I can prove, universal validity of this or any information. In the previous chapter I made mention of mystic intellectuals who have had a severe impact on the realm of the intellect today. I have also stated that these, as many of today's so called experts of science and philosophy, have had a hand in disintegrating man's certainty of universal truths in our culture; a culture that is morally-intellectually bankrupt. A culture that has been misguided and demoralized by those whose profession is to provide rational guidance: the professional intellectuals—our university professors and philosophers. Where is the evidence of this you ask? Just look around you, at the stature of our country today, and how America is literally dying.

The economy has been struck hard and we are on the verge of another great depression; the government is now bigger today then at any other point in American history and is still growing; freedom of speech, the last leg of a free society, is on the threshold of eradication!—why? Why has America descended into the nadir ring of hell, spun off the glory that it once held so highly and righteously over the despotic civilizations of the past? It is for the reason that this is where the *experts*, today's modern and postmodern philosophers and their intellectual progeny, have guided us. Perpetuated through today's rapid disintegration, abnegation and abrogation of individual rights, of reason, i.e., of the Constitution and the bill of right for which the greatest country in history was founded upon…all being replaced by the rapid employment of a fascist government. The intellectuals and politicians of today preach, and I do mean literally preach in the same fashion and within the same context as priests, that there is no law of causality and every governmental action must be taken on faith.

They assert, in reason's stead, anti-causality, the reverse of specific causes resulting in specific effects. That having the effect will somehow grant them the virtue of the cause. Observable with the belief that having the government promiscuously increasing the number of jobs without the businessmen's commercial demand will somehow increase economic productivity or that implementing a minimum wage or increasing pay without an employee showing the ability worth an increase will somehow cause an increase in the employee's efficacy and national wealth. A trend of thought that has bled its way into bodybuilding with the belief that increasing muscular size and strength will somehow grant you the virtue of being healthy and a goal-oriented, diligent, efficacious being...but more often than not results in many individuals turning to the use of dangerous quantities of steroids and other growth promoting substances...individuals who stand blind in the dark hallway of the world with their hand on the light switch of reason, but they instead reach for the glow of an arching current in a puddle of water. Such irrational premises are the reason why today's generation of scholars that our universities are releasing into the world are intellectually-morally bare of defenses, possessing the self-destructive shackles of an irrational philosophy that they have accepted as the only truth; naked in the world with no means of telling truth from falsehood, right from wrong. What is right and what is wrong?—blank out. Their irrational-mystic-subjective ethos asserts that nothing is ultimately true and nothing is ultimately false, that knowledge is a false perception; that 2+2=4 today, but it may equal 3.5 or 4 million tomorrow.

Even Physicists (the most admired strata of intellectuals of all time) have degraded into a mass, or a non-mass (having no value, for those not literate in physics terminology), of nonsensical subjective whim worshipping. Examples like the French physicists Igor and Grichka Bogdanov, who presented a lecture of their speculations about the universe before the Big Bang that left their colleagues in a state of utter disbelief. Their colleagues were faced with two alternatives: either this was some parody of contemporary cosmology or these brothers were damn serious. The truth of the matter was that they were completely serious. The result of this was that their colleagues felt forced to admit to the public that much of the research presented today is indistinguishable from a joke.

You ask what relevance does this have in bodybuilding. Everything! Bodybuilding does not exist within a vacuum. The viral moral and intellectual deprivation of our intellectuals has an unprecedented affect on the ideas of any individual who seeks physical magnificence, by means of undercutting the facility that is his only tool capable of allowing him to acquire the knowledge necessary to reach his muscular goals. If you are honestly pursuing the actualization of your physique aspirations, the development of your mind must be the first and foremost concern of your efforts, as it is vitally imperative in your potential of success over failure, of muscle growth over muscular atrophy, of life over death!

In this chapter, I will be dealing with the fundamental philosophic principles of reality that will enable you to gain the fundamental foundation indispensable in your understanding of, not just bodybuilding exercise science, but all of the sciences…at least the fundamentals of objective scientific theories.

Why is it that a book on bodybuilding is dedicated to the focus of philosophy? It is because philosophy is extraordinarily important. It is, as Ayn Rand said, the wholesaler of man's affairs: the most powerful force in human life. Everybody has a philosophy. However, what philosophy you have is a matter of choice, and most people do not make a conscious choice with regard to what philosophy they accept. Their philosophies become merely a grab-bag of arbitrary, disconnected and contradictory notions erratically absorbed from television, newspapers, books, family, religion and the like. As a result, their philosophies are an intellectually encumbering chaos of contradictions....A philosophy full of contradictions can prove to be very lethal.

I have aspired to show you just how important a rational philosophy is in the efficacy of your life—intellectually, emotionally and physically. However, since I do not believe that anyone has the right to force another individual to do anything or to believe anything, nor do I believe anyone should take someone on blind faith. I hold that, *it is only on the basis of grasping an argument that one should agree or not*, including the subject of bodybuilding. And bodybuilding, just as all things man encounters in life, has a philosophy...however, with all of the conflicting training methods and theories, bodybuilding—just as all of today's intellectual realms—have people possessing differing philosophic views on the subject.

But understand that just because someone has a philosophy on how to conduct their efforts does not make it correct or even slightly valid. There is only one reality and therefore there can only be one immutable and ultimately correct philosophy that coincides with it. And it is the philosophy behind the theory of high intensity training, though, that I affirm with scientific correctitude and empirical substantiation, is the only correct and objective (i.e. universally valid) theory of bodybuilding exercise science. However, since I have no right to force you to believe this nor do I expect you to take me on blind faith, I will explain fundamentally why the theory of high intensity training is valid by illuminating the means by which man acquires his knowledge of the absolutes of the universe. In order to do this I must explain by what means man discovers objective truth and how he is able to form a universally valid answer for any subject within reality—I must explain the fundamentals of a rational philosophy.

First of all, many people are confused about what exactly is philosophy...most think of it as sort of intellectual tomfoolery of people who have too much time on their hands. I can honestly say that when I was younger, my perception of what a philosopher was consisted of nothing more than an individual talking nonsense like a homeless man on the street corner proclaiming that the end is near and trying to tell me that the meaning of life was something that only he knew due to some unworldly endowment...which only goes to show that I was quite a perceptive child. But I was completely blind to the true vital value of philosophy since a smokescreen of fools and psychopaths presented philosophy under a disgusting false pretense of mysticism and obedience to something...whether it was a god, the government or anyone else, I did not take kindly to someone attacking my freedom to live my dreams.

Most, nearly all save for a very rare few, philosophers teach absolutely nothing of value...nothing relevant to reality and the truth. If you have found yourself dumbfounded by the gibberish that you hear in a philosophy class, you are not alone. Of course it is difficult to try to listen to someone telling you to act against everything that your senses have told you up to now...in the very same way that shooting yourself in the leg is preceded by every alarm signal in your head yelling stop!

Philosophy is the subject that studies *man's* relationship to reality, neither man apart from reality nor reality apart from man as many of today's accepted philosophers would have you believe. Philosophy is man's means of understanding and of evaluating values, ideas, morality and his identity in the universe. Whether you reject philosophy or not, you are of the species man and, because of which, you possess a *specific* method of self-sustaining action. "In order to live, man must act; in order to act, he must make choices; in order to make choices, he must define a code of values; in order to define a code of values, he must know *what* he is and *where* he is—*i.e.*, he must know his own nature (including his means of knowledge) and the nature of the universe in which he acts—*i.e.*, he needs metaphysics, epistemology, ethics, which means: *philosophy*. He cannot escape from this need; his only alternative is whether the philosophy guiding him is to be chosen by his mind or by chance." (Ayn Rand, "Philosophy and Sense of Life," *The Romantic Manifesto*)

Philosophy has two cardinal branches: *Metaphysics* and *Epistemology*. Flowing from them are three evaluative branches of philosophy: Ethics, Politics and Esthetics, all of which are entwined in framework of this book and a complete examination of all of philosophy is far beyond the scope of this work—but if you are interested I suggest that you read Ayn Rand's radical, thought provoking novel *Atlas Shrugged*.

The first nine chapters of this book are structured around the subject of metaphysics and epistemology, in the last two chapters I will be focusing on the metaphysical nature of man's survival discovered through epistemology: ethics. In this chapter, I will only be focusing only on the philosophic fundamentals that are the foundation that will allow you to become able to grasp the fundamental principles of the universe (metaphysics), which will allow you to grasp most, if not all, of the future facts of physics and human physiology to be presented, and man's method of survival (epistemology).

Reality

Metaphysics is the fundamental branch of philosophy that makes everything else in philosophy possible. Metaphysics is the branch of philosophy that studies the nature of the universe as a whole, in essence, reality. Fundamentally, metaphysics is the study of three axiomatic concepts: existence, consciousness and identity. Metaphysics is the branch of philosophical study that all bodybuilders should become acquainted with if they are to fully grasp the nature of muscle's power to increase in size and strength, and the fact that such a result is not unique and unknowable, but universal and comprehensible.

The first axiom, existence, is elucidated by the objective fact that *existence* exists—existence is absolute! This axiom does not tell us anything about the nature or the identity of existence, but merely the fact that it exists. This axiom is the foundation of everything else in philosophy. Before you are capable of asking what things there are or what problems man faces in understanding them there must first **be** something. In grasping any further knowledge of why or how to building larger muscles, there must exist the entity man and the entity muscle.

However, to be capable of questioning what things there are or even to understand them there must first be a consciousness to question and comprehend. The second axiom consciousness is the faculty of awareness, of that which exists. It perceives reality by integrating its sensory perceptions of reality into percepts. If there is no reality, there cannot be a consciousness. A consciousness perceives reality; it does not create it. A consciousness only conscious of itself is a contradiction in terms. In order for a consciousness to be conscious of something there must first **be** something to be conscious of.

The third and final axiom, identity, is a corollary of the axiom existence. To exist is to be something. To be something *is* to have identity to differentiate it from nothingness; whether that something is an object, an action or a characteristic: *existence is identity*, as Ayn Rand stated. The axiom identity does not deal with the fact that something exists, but merely the fact that something that exists is itself.

"Whatever you choose to consider, be it an object, an attribute or an action, the law of identity remains the same. A leaf cannot be a stone at the same time, it cannot be all red and all green at the same time, it cannot freeze and burn at the same time. A is A. Or, if you wish it stated in simpler language: You cannot have your cake and eat it, too." (John Galt's Speech, *Atlas Shrugged*)

The absolute proof that the law of identity contributes in validating the universal appositeness of the theory of high intensity training is that to be something in existence is to have a specific nature or an identity. To have an identity is to have characteristics or aspects unique to it; A is A—a thing is itself. I quote from a speech that I conducted at training and nutritional seminar that explains identity's necessity in the field of exercise science.

"Some people will still come up to me with the

uneducated response that 'everyone is different [because of which] nothing applies to everyone'.

"These people do not understand the concept of identity. They denote illogical concepts of, 'if I don't want something to be it won't.' The idea that everyone's muscles respond to different stimuli is exactly akin to stating that, that rock there will fall when I drop it, but that rock beside it will not do the same. These people lack a grasp of the concept of reality, [that is] of existence, of identity. As Aristotle implicitly stated, A is A; and this is universal as A can only be A, and muscle can only be muscle. If *a* muscle requires a high intensity stimuli to hypertrophy (i.e. to grow) then all muscles require it, because A is A.

"If everyone was different in the way that these people claim, there would not be a medical science. If everyone's cells, organs, and tissues were constituted and functioned differently, then none of the medical techniques used successfully thousands of times everyday by doctors around the world would work. If everyone is different and nothing is applicable to everyone then there cannot be a universal approach to neither proper medicine nor surgery, as every person on earth would require a special doctor just for them."

*   *   *

The universal import of the three axioms are that they are the primary non-reducible means of identifying everything within the universe—the universe being everything that exists—and the only means of correctly judging the true validity of concepts and theories. The *axiomatic concepts are the guardians of man's mind and the foundation of reason.*

The axioms are *self-evident* truths of the universe that are unable to be analyzed (i.e. proven) or broken up into component parts, as they are our *primary* means of identifying and analyzing that which exists. They are the primary implicit concepts that are our means, the foundation, of concept-formation. They are "primary implicit" concepts for the reason that they are always available to your consciousness, but are that which you have and have not yet conceptualized: they are the three fundamentals of everything in the universe—all that man has dealt with, is currently dealing with and has yet to deal with.

To try to disprove them is self-contradictory, as you would be trying to disprove them by using the axioms as your method of disproving them. The three axioms have, to quote Dr. Leonard Peikoff, "a built-in protection against all attacks: they must be used and accepted by everyone, including those who attack them and those who attack the concept of the self-evident." For instance, if someone were to tell you, "Existence doesn't exist", they would be automatically stating that *existence* exists, for the reason that reality is an absolute. If nothing existed there would be no question of its existence—who would question it?

If someone were to state that, "Man is an unconsciousness being", they would be accepting consciousness, because if man had no consciousness how could he form the question of its existence? Feelings are incapable of forming concepts and abstractions…by what means does a "non-autonomous man", to quote the dimwitted B.F Skinner, form vocal and written communication and long-range goals?

Finally, if someone were to state, "Just because some theory is true for you, does not mean it is true for me. [That is] all people who disagree about the identity of the very same point are equally, objectively correct". Their statement, though denouncing absolutism of the law identity, is conceding to identity: they are using symbols (i.e. words) that possess the identity of specific concepts that possess *a* specific referent to a metaphysical concrete—referring to the same entity, characteristic or action before everyone's consciousness. Furthermore, if two concepts contradict each other they both cannot be right; A is A. If you are to state that existents do not have identity, that is to say, that they are not themselves, then you are stating that nothing exists since *existence is identity*.

One question asked of me, based on the inquiry of all three axioms, was, "How do you really know if we all perceive the same reality. Individuals possess different degrees of ocular capability, with some individuals that are color blind and others that can apparently see strings of color while listening to music differing from the norm." Well it is actually true that we all do see different degrees of color. Neuroscientists have proven recently that the number of color-sensitive cones in the retina differ dramatically among individuals. So as a result, the degree of redness of an object has that you perceive is different than mine, yet that does not change the fact that we still perceive the same entity and its identity presenting the color red, no matter who views it. Neuroscience shows that the brain controls our perception of color more than our eyes, since the eyes are merely a lens that fires neurons when exposed to a spectrum of light waves and it is the job of the brain to bring forth an image amid the flood of neural data.

Such things as color blindness and perceiving colors while listening to music do not represent different realities or an ability to view an esoteric reality over the norm. Color blindness is a genetic defect or contagion/ trauma pathology in the eye (such as a complete lack of one or two of the three types of the light sensitive cones in the eye), an abnormality in the neural pathways from the retina to the brain, or a defect in the proper function of the brain in translating neural data. A condition that is diagnosed by identifying specific parts of the visual system that are *malfunctioning*—just as with kidneys, a pathology, like chronic renal failure, means that the body of some individual who possess such conditions do not function properly—they depart from their intended function, resulting in a lesser than favorable outcome. They do not come to the realization of their true "individual" functional nature.

The ability to see colors while listening to music, also known as Synesthesia, is a rare neurologically based phenomenon in which the stimulation of one sensory organ (like the ear) can involuntarily and automatically activate another part of the brain that creates images and have one seeing strings of vibrant color while hearing a symphony.

Now, some self-arrested people will still implore you to prove the existence of the axioms. This, of course, is a stupid question; to quote Dr. Leonard Peikoff, "There is only one answer to this: stop the discussion. Axioms *are* self-evident; no argument can coerce a person who chooses to evade them."

To try to prove the existence of the axioms is self-contradictory, as you would be trying to prove existence by the standard of non-existence or consciousness by the standard of unconsciousness. You are essentially regarding *nothing* as an entity, as a something that exists, and trying to prove that something exists by stating that it exists merely because it is a non-nothing or a non-zero.

This of course is absurd, since the concept of non-existence is only relevant if you first grasp that something exists, and then realize that when it is absent from existence that there is a non-existence. Non-existence is not an entity, it is a zero with no potential, it has no identity. Someone insisting that you prove the existence of the axioms is telling you to step into an abyss outside of existence and consciousness to prove their validity. He is, as Ayn Rand stated, asking you to become a zero gaining knowledge about a zero.

The only method in which you can prove their existence is by means of ostensive evidence—using examples, directly perceivable by the body's sensory organs, of the thing you are trying to prove. To prove existence, look around you and observe this book, a chair, a table—they *exist*. To prove consciousness, pinch yourself, do you notice a sensation—you are *conscious* of it. To prove identity, examine the content of this book or the shape of a chair or the size of a table—they have *identity*. You can only prove the axioms by perceiving examples of them directly. Just try to explain to an individual who was born blind what the magnificence of New York City looks like at night. A City with a melodic intensity of a medium of steel, concrete and shimmering rivers of glass—cut with straight lines and angles, all painted with a composition of electronic brilliant color and dramatic shades realized by the potential of man's mind and his free will. Or try to explain to someone who was born deaf what romantic and emotionally stirring power a masterpiece such as Frederick Chopin's Nocturne in C# minor has on a passionately driven individual…you can't, there are no functional direct sensational examples to demonstrate there existence or identity.

The Law of Causality

The law of causality is the corollary of the axiom identity. The law of causality, to quote Ayn Rand, is the law of identity applied to action. Whereas, the law of identity dictates that you cannot have your cake and eat it too, the law of causality dictates that you cannot eat your cake before you have it.

All actions are caused by entities. The nature of an action is determined by the nature of the entity that acts; a thing cannot act in contradiction to its nature, as Aristotle stated with his recognition of the law of noncontradictory identification. A muscle is a muscle is a muscle and its nature dictates that it requires a specific cause to be stimulated into the desired effect of growth. The same absolutism applies to you if you were to jump off the edge of the cliff. Because of the nature of the gravitational pull of the earth and its effect on your body, when there is nothing to oppose your body's downward force (cause) you *will* plummet towards the ground (effect), and rather quickly I might add. …Feel free to ignore and dispute it all you like, but I will not be the one to clean up the mess you leave behind, or as Alan Sokal said after the example he set with the postmodern cultural studies journal *Social Text*, "Anyone who believes that the laws of physics are mere social conventions is invited to try transgressing those conventions from the windows of my apartment. (I live on the twenty-first floor.)."

When a child reaches the stage of (implicitly) grasping the concepts entity, identity, and action, he possesses the requisite knowledge to understand (implicitly) the law of causality. To take this step the child needs to observe an omnipresent truth: that an entity of a specific kind acts in a specific manner—that a thing is its self and acts accordingly. The child learns this by observing that when he performs a specific action on a specific entity that a specific action is brought forth—e.g., when he shakes his rattle a noise is produced, but when he shakes a wooden block, it does not produce a noise. The child comes to (implicitly) grasp that a specific entity is the *cause* of a specific effect and that actions (his shaking an entity in this instance) do not produce actions; only entities produce actions.

The law of causality is the universal law of reality, that nothing within the universe occurs causeless—some specific *entity* produces some specific *result*. Ayn Rand stated it definitively when she stated in *Philosophy: Who Needs It*, "Since things are what they are, since everything that exists possesses a specific identity, nothing in reality can occur causelessly or by chance."

The law of causality rests on two points: that action is action of an entity; and the law of identity, that things are what they are, A is A. With this premise we know that all entities have a specific, noncontradictory, nature that is limited; it possesses specific attributes and no others—that is to say, *it must act in accordance with its nature.*

This being true, we are able to identify specific causes resulting in effects of an entity, devoid of a caprice nature that would be impossible to study, to predict, to know. A universe not governed by the universal law of cause and effect would be utter chaos. Such things impossible to image such as gorilla shaped apples materializing out of thin air and exploding with the force of a billion atomic bombs would not be possible or impossible, how would we know if they were or not. Since there would be no specific causes, breathing could result in pregnancy or even a PhD (though the latter seems to be the case nowadays). Now you, at the very least, come to grasp the utter absurdity of philosophers that state there are no causes to effects—furthermore, why our economy seems to be "plummeting off the edge of a cliff" as the government ignores the lethal effects of their actions, declaring that the ends *unconditionally* justifies the means, when they ignore the fact that socialism didn't work in Russia, it didn't work in England and it will not work in the United States or Canada, I promise you that.

Now since our primary concern as bodybuilders is to build big muscles we require a conceptual grasp of the cause and effect relationship of the stimulus and the circumstances that results in a compensator buildup of muscular size and strength. However, in order to grasp such an abstract concept as muscle growth we require an understanding of how or even if man can gain such knowledge—we must become familiar with the nature of thought itself.

Thought

*"Facts are stubborn things; and whatever
may be our wishes, our inclinations, or the
dictates of our passions, they cannot alter
the state of facts and evidence."*

John Adams, the Second
President of the United States

Epistemology is the branch of philosophy that studies the nature and means of human knowledge; dedicated to discovering the proper method of acquiring and validating knowledge, in effect, the study of reason. The foundation of all of man's knowledge is acquired by means of his awareness through his sensory perception of reality. Unlike animals, man is not an instinctual creature, he is a *conceptual* being—he deals with and survives by the abstractions and concepts that he (cognitively) constructs from his sensory information.

Every living species on earth must pursue a specific course of action in order to survive, and its specific course of action is dictated by its *nature*. The course of action that is required for man's survival is first and foremost an intellectual one. His method of survival is his mind.

Man's mind, just as his body and everything else that exists, possesses a *specific* nature. Man is born defenseless with no readily available physical means of defending or feeding himself. He "has no claws, no fangs, no horns, no great strength of muscle. He must plant his food or hunt it. To plant, he needs a process of thought. To hunt, he needs weapons, and to make weapons—a process of thought." (Howard Roark's trial speech, *The Fountainhead*)

Though man's mind is given to him at birth, its content is not; man is born "tabula rasa." The only way man can survive is by his faculty of reason. If he does not use reason as his guide of pursuing valid knowledge of reality, he dies. Man's senses are his only direct cognitive contact with reality and, therefore, his *only* source of information to which reason is required for understanding. However, reason does not work automatically. Man must make the consistent and ever active *volitional* effort to use reason. Man's sensatory perceptions of reality, via his sight, touch, taste, hearing and smell, are integrated from sensations into percepts involuntary and automatically; senses that tell him that something *is*, but not what it *is*—only his mind can do that. The specific manner for which man's mind uses his precepts to gain valid knowledge is not involuntary or automatic.

Man's mind is man's mind and must acquire knowledge of reality by specific means (reason) in accordance with specific rules (logic). And logic is logic—there is no Aryan logic, no poly logic, no feminist logic, no democratic logic; there is only the logic of the species man and logic (the art of non-contradictory identification) is man's method, his only method, of reaching *objective* conclusions by deriving them without contradiction from the facts of reality (ultimately, from the evidence provided by his senses). Thus, logic rests on the metaphysical axioms that existence exists and existence is identity. Man's knowledge is not acquired by logic apart from empirical evidence (experience) nor by the empirical apart from logic, but by the employment of logic to the empirical. Thus, all truths are the product of a logical identification of the facts of experience.

However, bear in mind that, in any hour and moment

of his life, man is free to choose to think logically, rationally or opt abdicate that effort. But he is not free to avoid the ramifications of his actions. Man has been defined as the "rational being", but rationality is a matter of *his* choice. Nature, the law of causality, leaves man with only two alternatives: rational being or suicidal animal; productive, efficacious being or cognitively abstained corpse; man or non-man.

If man chooses rationality—rationality being the acknowledgment of the fact that existence exists; that reality is immutable and that nothing can alter the truth; that nothing can take precedence over that act of perceiving it, which is thinking—he must make the conscious and unremitting effort to use reason has his *only* means of judging information and gaining his knowledge. If man chooses to be rational "most" of the time and is irrational only some of the time, when it suits him, he abandons his moral integrity, permitting irrationality the same conceptual validity as rationality. He is thus abdicating his mind by accepting the supernatural as an absolute and thereby, consciously or unconsciously, rejecting the absolutism of reality and reason—damning is means of survival. As John Galt stated so eloquently in Atlas Shrugged, "If you compromise food with poison, it is only death that can win."

A man of such an intellectual-emotional dichotomy cannot function properly—growing continuously uncertain of what is the right or the wrong, the true or the untrue, the pro-life or the pro-death, to the degree that he holds irrationalities as being valid. He stands panic-stricken; his irrational convictions oppose his rational ones, resulting in uncertainty. The man becomes split in two. He franticly seeks whatever mystical-subjective ethics he has accepted or is being drawn to by default, but cries in agony over the emotional torment he has inherently accepted for reasons that he cannot explain, unable to fully grasp the irrational…the mystic. He becomes torn between the practical (that which allows man his survival) and the moral (the good, that which allows man self-esteem).

In order for man to progress by gaining and keeping his values—ultimately, his life—he must think and pursue valid non-contradictory knowledge. If man arrives at a contradiction he has made an error in his thinking and has the capability to reexamine the issue and correct it. But to maintain a contradiction in the context of one's mind is to abdicate one's mind and detach oneself from reality. The moral principle that is paramount to an individual's psychological and existential wellbeing is an uncompromising moral integrity and judgment. The acceptance of the fact that reality *is* black and white—there is no moral or metaphysical grayness—and that to abstain from moral judgment in a *moral* issue (including that of the intellect), proclaiming an issue to being "middle-of-the-road" or neither right nor wrong only a shade of gray is to promote the wrong, the evil, by not punishing it. In addition to condemning the right, the good, by not rewarding it with the payment it earned. The outcome of a middle-of-the-roader or one who abdicates moral judgment under the premise of everything just being a shade of grayness, if uncorrected, is moral bankruptcy and intellectual abandonment by default…sound familiar?

Now, since man gains and holds his knowledge in conceptual form, the validity of man's knowledge depends on the validity of his concepts, i.e., the precision of their definitions. To quote Ayn Rand, from *Introduction to Objectivist Epistemology*, "Since concepts, in the field of cognition, perform a function similar to that of numbers in the field of mathematics, the function of a proposition is similar to that of an equation: it applies conceptual abstractions to a specific problem.

"A proposition, however, can perform this function only if the concepts of which is composed have precisely defined meanings. If, in the field of mathematics, numbers had no fixed, firm values, if they were approximations determined by the mood of their users—so that "5," for instance, could mean five in some calculations, but 61/2 or 43/4 in others, according to the user's 'convenience'— there would be no such thing as mathematics."

Realize that human knowledge has a nature, and man's knowledge is hierarchical in structure, with every higher-level concept being based on lower level, less abstract and more concrete, information. Higher level abstractions or derivatives such as whether to use a wide-grip or close-grip for pulldowns or whether it is better to perform regular or stiff leg deadlifts, though important, have no significance until you grasp the fundament principles which permit these supplementary considerations to be worthy of beneficial deliberation.

Just as when we are dealing with mathematical science. In mathematics you require specific fundamental knowledge to grasp and deal with further abstract and complex equations; the fundamental principles being addition, subtraction, multiplication and division. To attempt to ascertain the complexities of abstract algebra or calculus without the mathematical fundamentals is to idle in an intellectual stupor.

* * *

If you are to find the cause for your current or past beliefs, moreover to discover the validity of them, you must understand how one acquires his knowledge: "Is this approach to building muscle the most productive?", "Where did I get this information from; can I trust it and is it based on the one arbiter of truth—reality?" These questions are the basis for which one can discover the method needed in their pursuit of a more productive training approach, as with everything else in life: *to always question why and how.*

If you are to carryout your bodybuilding efforts in the most efficacious manner possible you must adhere to reason, there is no other alternative—*reason is absolute*. If you are pursuing a training method or anything else in life and come to a contradiction, check your premises. Keep in mind Aristotle's law of identity, reality has no contradictions, so go back through the hierarchy of your current knowledge and find the flaw(s). Once finding the flaw you must evaluate and correct the mistake by means of weighing it against reality...the truth. If you were using reason as your means of discovering truth you will find it simple and very rewarding to correct the mistake by retracing your mental steps back to its concrete foundation, you may even discovery something that you were not looking for, but becomes extremely useful in your future efforts, as has been the case with much of my research.

Philosophical Application of Reason to Today's Intellectual Crisis

"If you believe everything you read, better not read."

Old Japanese Proverb

When man judges by means of *his* faculty of reason, that is to say, judgment founded upon the three fundamental axioms of the universe, their derivatives and the adherence to their absolutism, man is able to discover objective truth (non-bias and incoercible to any form of thought, wish or non-existent spiritual zero—being universally valid). Reality is the ultimate arbiter of the truth. However, this does not mean that man is incapable of judging the truth for himself nor does it mean that his judgment is omniscient or infallible—it only dictates his means of finding objective truth: logic.

If you are in doubt in regards to the validity of the theory of high intensity training, the greatest method of finding the truth is to look for its referents—i.e., to ask oneself: what fact or facts of reality gave rise to this theory? Are there any contradictions or unintelligible user exceptions with the theory's practice (i.e. invalid for certain ages, genders, or only producing results for a minority of individuals, etc.)?

If it is individuality that you desire, then undertake the intimately individual endeavor of thinking for yourself. Judge for *yourself*—not by tradition, religion or majority vote whether something is morally acceptable for you to believe, pursue and perform—use your reason. Thought is one of the most personally intimate and selfish acts that one can perform—that can only be performed by the mind of the individual. There is no such thing as a "collective mind," only a group of individuals, each being capable of independent thought, but making decisions as the result of a collective vote. However, to live by majority consensus, one abdicates their mind and their life to whim of the potentially stupid and those who may believe they have the "right" to the effort and the property of others…that is, believing that they possess the right to the minds and livelihood of other individuals.

If you desire to know the truth *you* are the one that must make the volitional effort to find it, whether someone has discovered it or not has no relevance as long you do not make the conscious effort to use your reason as a means to find, understand and appreciate the value of their discovery. And doing so today is a more demanding task than ever—though well worth the work for those who seek efficacy in their training, nutrition, business, intellectual independence and happiness.

There are many who will attempt to make you accept their beliefs on merit of pure faith—faith being a complete *blind* trust in someone or something in the absence of or in direct contradiction to evidence. But, whether these faith-based assertions are those of your teachers, politicians or even your parents *you must not take them on faith*…not if you are to discover truth and live a rational life where you recognize that effects have causes, that the universe can be understood, but only through rational thought and not by faith.

Your only means to defend yourself against such intellectual cowards, looters, and destroyers of other men's achievements and vehement despisers of man's mind, who dismiss the absolutism of specifically caused effects or just disregard their absolutism as having nothing to do with reality, is *your* mind. To protect yourself you cannot think with an open-mind, giving everything said, written or televised as having some truth as many naysayers of certainty will tell you, but neither with a closed-mind that attempts to reject those who spew nonsense and inimical advice, because you will also inadvertently reject those who speak the truth. Your only method to wade through today's ocean of the mystical-emotionalist-subjectivist junk heap, separating truth from falsehood, is to *think critically*, in an ever-active pursuit of the right over the wrong by man's means of discovering truth (logic).

Thinking critically is not to deeming every piece of information with automatically none or some validity… nor is it just leaving it in some contextual amoral grayness in your subconscious. Thinking critically is to call forth reason on tribunal and having reality as the judge to the validity of the information. No, learning to think logically and to judge critically is not easy, but neither is bodybuilding.

The most active manner of critical thinking of the information people present is to take everything said by them *literally* and judge it by the ramifications of what was said if pursued in reality. Many people will defend with such common retaliations as that was not what they really meant to say or you are taking it the wrong way and just don't understand what they really mean…. Oh really? If that is not what they meant to say then why did they say it? And if it was a mistake of communicating what they really meant why do they insist on reiterating it, and further, to continue inculcating others to it, not correcting the mistake(s) he made? And if I do not understand what they really mean why don't you explain? Why were they incapable of explaining it in a way that every rational individual can understand by using demonstrable evidence in reality? Why…and how?

One must come to realize that words are a very powerful tool. The likes of which that have the potential to teach man the wonders of the world, from such wondrous things as the stunning complexities and wondrous intricacies of galaxies to the intimate ballet of subatomic particles in atoms, while sitting in his living room. They have the power to motivate men with a way of communicating their efficacy and passion as thinking beings. A medium of communication that can motivate others who fuel his motivation by sharing discoveries and interests in common values—the power to allow man to learn from his mistakes or to avoid past mistakes by reading about the past errors of ancient civilizations to modern economic relationships. However, words also have the power, when the reader does not seriously evaluate the validity of the information, to disintegrate man's mind and instill self-despisal and intellectual uncertainty. Religion, Platonism in the intellectual realm, is the original proprietor of today's self-questioning and self-destruction, and the main influence of today's intellectual black hole. Religion is anti-man, that is to say, against man's means of survival.

Many individuals will retort in contempt that religion has brought order to man in face of anarchy. But such responses are to be expected from those who are inundated with false premises and history presented through rose-colored glasses. Recall such destruction and atrocities on the body and the mind as the Roman Inquisition, the witch-hunts of the 1600s, the Aztec human sacrifices, the Christian Crusades, or the Islamic Jihads, to name but a tiny fraction of an extensive list. Religion—true religion as was the rule in the dark ages—is only a semiorganized anarchy with appointed mystics who point to who will be the next victims, creating a different arena, one of semi-indiscriminate massacres, but with "bonus" of murderers having a "moral" or "righteous" sanction to their actions by the so-called messenger of god at that time. And it is again the resurgence of religion that has all but destroyed our once free country...well not yet. Religion though had made a compromise over 200 years ago in order for it to survive the industrial revolution, which followed from the enlightenment.

Religion had to do so under all periods of advancements of man—no matter how brief they were: the golden ages of Ancient Greece, the birthplace of reason; the Renaissance with Thomas Aquinas resurrecting Aristotelian logic back from the dark ages; the Enlightenment with the founding fathers that gave rise to the freest country in the world that broke free of the bondages of servitude and made possible the greatest triumph of man's history, the industrial revolution. All advancements of man, all technological, economic, social developments of man to this point today was brought forth, not by a faith in religion, not by faith in society, but through an understanding and adherence to reason, by personal ambition of individuals desiring to realize a dream. When man was finally released from the shackles of tyranny and monarchy rule, the industrial revolution brought forth the greatest success of man to date. But then came along the philosophy of a German philosopher that set his eyes on the task of disintegrating the intellect and returning morality to the province of the mystics. The main cause of today's intellectual-moral disintegration and our fast return to the dark ages is principally the work of one man: Immanuel Kant.

The Requiem of Man's Right to Life, Liberty and the Pursuit of Happiness

> *"Religious bondage shackles and debilitates the mind and unfits it for every noble enterprise....During almost fifteen centuries has the legal establishment of Christianity been on trial. What have been its fruits? More or less, in all places, pride and indolence in the clergy; ignorance and servility in laity; in both, superstition, bigotry, and persecution."*

James Madison, the Fourth
President of the United States

Though I will not go into comprehensive detail, I will state the decisive factor that made Immanuel Kant the seed that erupted into the deceitful canopy of uncertainty that darkened the light of truth with the murkiness of its shade. The likes of which that is the cause of today's intellectual and moral down spiral. Immanuel Kant was able to penetrate the industrious and rational guidance of the early American sense of life by disguising his philosophy under the guise of the title "pure reason," when in fact Kant was the antithesis of reason. Kant brought back *pure* religion, devoid of its pagan elements, in the disguise of that which drew man from religion to create the greatest country the world had ever seen—reason.

While Plato and the medievalists of the churches

denied existence in the name of a castle in the sky, a super-reality, in which they believed they were in direct inspiring contact. Kant denied existence, not in the name of a fantasy, but of nothingness. Platonist, the mystics, believed that this mystic realm could be approached by the mind, even though they believe the mind is tainted by the body. That man should sacrifice his earthy desires, but do so for the sake of gaining a reward in the next life: their proper goal was happiness, though not in this life. Kant on the other hand proclaimed that man's proper goal, in Kant's words, is not happiness, whether in this life or the next. But that the "radically evil creature," as Kant referred to man, should sacrifice his desires from duty—holding duty as an end in itself.

Kant proclaimed that man has no right to his life and must *sacrifice* himself to justify his existence, i.e., he must sacrifice his values that are essential to him for a lesser or non-value—and the greater the value the greater the sacrifice. Whether the sacrifice is the food off his table in favor of those who did not earn it, but demanded their "right" to his food. Or the shirt off his back to those who refuse to earn it, but demanded those who did to keep them alive from the elements. Or his children to those who have none, but demanded his in the name of "fairness" to the barren and the infertile, to the sacrifice of a woman's body to the *potential* child that she has no financial ability to care for nor desire to parent. A control that the politicians now possess that demands that she give-up her life, her aspiration and her body in the name of something that they have the audacity to call prolife… such a violent hate of individual rights is the result of Kantian ethics. All ultimately leading to the sacrifice of his life to those who do not make an effort to live theirs, but demand that those who do are evil, that those of ability who worked for their own wealth and happiness, those *selfish* individuals, must serve the impotent. Kant held that, "happiness is not an ideal of reason, but of imagination." You say that such an end is not true? Then why don't just you ask one of the proletariats of the former Soviet Union what was going on behind that iron curtain.

Kant's philosophy was used as an umbrella of solace and sanction for those who exerted no effort to earn their life's goals, but sat in bewilderment of why they could not achieve them. For those who acted to the contrary of what their perceptions and rational thoughts told them was the truth, like Dostoevsky's Underground Man who cries: "What do I care for the laws of nature and arithmetic, when, for some reason, I don't like them, or the fact that two plus two equals four." People who became despondent and grew fiercely jealous of other individuals' material wealth, ability and happiness… people that looked to Kantian philosophy in a twisted delusion of a two-way-mirror that had them protected from the competent. A mirror that was inscribed with the proclamation that no man has the right to pursue his happiness…that it is his duty, according to his ability, to serve others—abdicating self-interest, self-esteem and pleasure to the impotent, the less fortunate, the deprived in order for one to be truly virtuous. But if one gained *any* return of pride, material reward, pleasure, or value of any kind it was not virtuous under Kant's morality.

Such a gelatinous society immersed in Kantian ethics is reinforced by his unintelligible metaphysical snare of,

"You can't know if you are right, your reality is not mine—the majority consensus agrees that this morality is true, who are you to question it?!" This is the parasitic paradise these people desired, where the able had to subordinate to the weak, the healthy to the sick, the passionate to the idle—a society that today is not being brought about by means of totalitarian force that was used in creating the USSR, but through our own sanction.

Kant's philosophy was and is used by those who demand that the productive, those of ability and self-sustaining drive, have no right to the product of their minds and that those of lesser ability and those who refuse to be productive have a moral right to it (… starting to sound quite familiar to today's politicians speeches, isn't it?). Kant damned the good for being the good—damning man for being man qua rational being. The results of such immoral, irrational premises lead to the gas chambers of Nazi Germany, the slave-labor camps of Soviet Russia, the brain drain of socialist England and the United States' current state of pandemonium.

Kantian and post-Kantian philosophy was, and still is, to an enormous degree, the dominate philosophy being taught at our collages and universities as the true theory of life for man, as the philosophy known as modernism, since the 19th century. But as of the mid 20th century even Kant's academic philosophy died along with the rest of the intellectuals whose worldview is disillusionment. He is dead, to quote Leonard Peikoff in his book *Objectivism: The Philosophy of Ayn Rand*, where nihilism, with little left to defy, is turning into its inevitable product: nihil (this is now being called 'minimalism' and 'postmodernism').

Though Kant's philosophy is dead, the momentum

of its destruction is still carrying our western civilization, not into a new dark age, as the consequence of Kantian ideology, but into an intellectual black hole (to quote Dr. Gary Hull). America has become a country devoid of ideology—a headless giant, staggering around in the dark towards a bottomless pit of rot, lead by the hand of faith (the antithesis of the original sin religion has damned man of—his mind) gripping tighter with every sanction of the bleeding victim to agree to the blade of some new unearned guilt that pulls him deeper and deeper into despair. The postmodern philosophers of today do not profess the need of philosophy or even try to understand the fundamentals of the mind or the universe. Today's philosophers condemn philosophy as having nothing to do with reality. Postmodernists promote nothing but pure passivity, that is to say, an avoidance of cultural argument. Consequently, they reject right and wrong and educate in our universities and public schools the practice of acting on pure emotions—on one's own, but more importantly, by a democratic vote how the majority feels.

We are taught not to be an "extremist" on any issue. In our schools we are told to give equal merit between all philosophies, cultural and political views. Between the opinions of everyone—not to give them just trail with your own moral judgment, but to completely abdicate judgment—save for a philosophy and political view that threatens this state of grayness and cultural confusion (which is why the consensus *blindly* rejects laissez-faire capitalism and a philosophy based on objective principles instead of vote, belief or feeling).

Our schools today teach moral *grayness*. They condemn and view "extremists," i.e. consistent individuals, as taking things "too" seriously or being closed minded to other possibilities—they despise the good for being pure and the evil for being tainted. The moral grayness that they advocate forgives the evil, as long as there is some good intention...what kind of good intention?—no response. Furthermore, it punishes the good for being good... what kind of good?—well how many children have been suspended or expelled for defending themselves in schools from bullies that physically threaten and enact harm and emotional torment, because they hurt the bully's "feelings" or caused him harm in defending themselves; how many University History and English classes reject the teachings of Shakespeare because feminists think of him as sexist or do not teach about Christopher Columbus discovering the new world that allowed man a taste of freedom for the first time in his history, because of the slavery of black Africans at the time. But worse than that, this moral grayness is little more than a hysterical revolt against reason and moral values, against absolutes.

They reward the atrocities of such things as the Rape of Nanking or the Rwanda Genocide with silence and obfuscation from the history books and say, "They are only human; let us forgive the murderers, the rapists, and the absolute racialist genocides." Such a reaction to such a degree of evil is revealing to the tyrants and terrorists of the world that there are no consequences for their acts of destruction; that the road is clear of obstruction and resistance—that their victims are tying their own hands taut and lashing their own backs so as not to inconvenience their "misunderstood" future despot.

Only a blind moron, and a suicidal one at that, believes that when an individual (bear in mind that a nation is only a sum of individuals) defends himself from the oppressive force of a bully, a tyrant, a murderer that he will be promoting further oppression. Avowing that the best thing to do is let the tyrant or bully have what he wants…that he will eventually become content and stop only ensures that the worst is yet to come (Czechoslovak comes to mind as a good example of the consequences of submitting to a tyrant). I quote Thomas Paine from his book *The Age of Reason*.

"Loving of enemies is another dogma of feigned morality, and has beside no meaning…. Those who preach the doctrine of loving their enemies are in general the greatest prosecutors, and they act consistently by so doing; for the doctrine is hypocritical, and it is natural that hypocrisy should act the reverse of what it preaches."

Postmodernists believe so strongly in the supremacy of emotions over reason that they openly support censorship of science and of free speech. For example, Professor Paul Feyerabend, formerly a professor of science at Berkley University, came out and openly indorsed the inquisition's enslavements of Galileo. Why you ask? Because the church at that time, argued Feyerabend, represented the community's "feelings." In his book "Farewell to Reason" Professor Feyerabend quoted, approvingly, Cardinal Robert Bellarmine, a 17th century theologian, who had condemned Galileo. "To affirm that the sun is at the center of the universe that only rotates on its axis, without going from east to west, is a very dangerous attitude, and one calculated to injure our faith by contradicting scriptures." Professor Feyerabend quoted this approvingly and then stated that "Galileo was as pushy and totalitarian as many profits of science and as uninformed. It is a pity that the church of today, frightened by the universal noise made by scientific wolves, prefers to howl with them *instead of trying to teach the scientists some manners.*" [Italics are mine]....That lone statement fittingly sums the current intellectual-moral bankruptcy of our culture. A bankruptcy that has begun escorting the cold, desolate hand of religion back into the intellectual void that our intellectuals have left behind, as has been the pattern of history's past.

*   *   *

Returning to a religious abstraction briefly for an abridgment and derision of religion, whether it is faith and worship of a god or today's worship and faith in "society." If some hypothetically omnipotent-omniscience entity, which does not live in the realm of reality, or the collective vote of the majority tells you that low intensity, high volume exercise will stimulate infinitely more muscle than brief and intense training, it does not have any capacity to make it so.

An entity that does not even live in the realm of reality—automatically making it a zero; a non-existent—, even if such a thing did exist, nor an infinity of eternities of desiring, wishing, praying or temper tantrums of fifty million Frenchmen has any power to alter reality. Why? Because A is A, muscle is muscle, a thing is itself and acts accordingly—owing to the fact that reality and the things that exist within it are objective not subjective. A thing will not change its or another entity's identity via mystical wish, prayer to some nonexistent mystical zero, or through blind ignorance of reason. *Reality is independent of consciousness*, i.e. objective. Remember, a consciousness perceives reality it does not form it or alter it.

To see the impotence of such philosophies of intellectual default and conduct based not on reason and empirical evidence, but on unquestioned feeling, aristocracy and faith one needs only to look at the history of man and how the experiments of such irrational and mystical philosophies defunct out. The foremost example of such for bodybuilding happened not too long ago.

In 1977, the famous docudrama Pumping Iron was released into theatres and the world was introduced to the intoxicating charisma and awe-inspiring physique of Arnold Schwarzenegger. With his breathtaking muscularity and a personality that commanded attention, Arnold made bodybuilding exciting, but he had his hand in today's current disintegration of it. Arnold, along with almost all bodybuilders at the time, explained that in order to obtain such muscular prowess you need to exercise… but that was more or less all that they explained. The young neophytic bodybuilders looked up to Arnold with the passionate hunger and observed that he and the other top rank bodybuilders lifted weights. When they asked the professionals what to do with these barbells and machines they were given a variation of three irrational answers: "Go by feeling, and use the 'instinctive' method of training"; "Do as I do, who are you to question my methods, who's the champion here?!"; and finally, "Just trying everything, everyone is different and needs different styles of training."

The result of this you ask? Well the size of the competitors at the professional level of bodybuilding grew…but that was only due to a greater number of individuals who took up bodybuilding—resulting in a greater pool of extremely genetically gifted individuals taking up bodybuilding. Yes there were more competitive bodybuilders on the scene, however, there were, and are now, hundreds of thousands of individuals who were and are unable to progress on such faith in the professionals and have given up in their goals or are still fruitlessly, blindly, running after it...running as fast as they can, unknowingly, in the opposite direction.

So after hearing the irrationalities and morally destructive ethos of today's culture, seeing that modern and postmodern philosophy has brought man to the lowest rung of hell, do we really need philosophy, if philosophy brought us to this point? Yes! Instead of seeing this as a sign of philosophy's impotence, one *must* distinguish this as the hallmark of philosophy's power over mankind—that one cannot treat the realm of ideas as recklessly and as foolishly as our intellectuals have been doing for far too long. Since man is man, A is A, and every living entity has a specific nature that dictates a specific course of action required for its survival; and since man's means of survival is ultimately his mind, philosophy is fundamental for every individual's success, development and, ultimately, survival. Every individual chooses a philosophy—whether they rigorously study and decide on one or unknowingly leave their subconscious to assemble an erratic, neurotic junk heap of a vague and arcane mongrel philosophy. Your success as a human being is dictated by the degree of your philosophical rationality. Reality rewards action founded on reason with success, pride, productivity, growth, life—the lesser of which one is consonant with reason, reality punishes man with failure, grief, confusion, incompetence, stagnation, death (and such penalties are his to bare alone).

To clarify the importance of philosophy in this book on bodybuilding, you must understand that man is an indivisible entity, an integrated unit of mind and body, to quote Mike Mentzer. What use is it for you to acquire the muscular physique of your dreams when you possess a mind that is distressingly riddled with confusion and uncertainty, unable to differentiate the good from the bad, the pro-life from the actions that lead to this inimical moral descent we are facing today? It is only by developing your mind through learning to think logically; acquiring the greatest power possible to man, not muscular power, but the power of the intellect—the power of *intellectual certainty*—that will allow you to be able to fully enjoy and appreciate the value of the fruits of your efforts, including that of achieving your full muscular potential. Remember, knowledge (truly valid ideas) is man's means of achieving all his goals, including that final goal or end which makes the others possible—the preservation and enhancement of his life.

This book is devoted and intended for the minority of individuals out there—no matter how small they maybe—who are tired of arbitrary pabulum of the subjective-mystic-traditionalism that our culture is drowning in. To the individuals who lust for more than there is now; individuals of intellectual and moral passion; the ones who question the majority, the politicians and the church, demanding that they answer *why* and *how* to their unintelligible culturally inculcated bromides—the individuals that hunger to see man as he might be, and ought to be, both physically and intellectually.

These are the individuals who will gain the most from these pages as they will receive the answers to the why's and how's of the body and of the mind. No, the information within this book is not an inexhaustible chasm of information, the likes of such detailed comprehension of every aspect of philosophy and bodybuilding is far beyond the scope of this work. If you have a desire to train your mind and gain an independent, objective, conceptual grasp of reality, I suggest you consider the works of Ayn Rand and Leonard Peikoff.

The structure and flow of the chapters ahead are presented in a manner to clarify general misconceptions on the subject and certain issues I present at the time—I will not dance around the deeper issues with unintelligible doubletalk, sometimes I will sound crude and I will be blunt, but such is only to present the matter as straightforward as possible without attempting to make you see the truth while wearing rose-colored glasses. My work is directed towards the few among the many, those who are tired of window-dressed incompetence and euphemized lies. So get ready, because, as the old saying goes, "You ain't seen nothing yet!"

Part II
The Science of Bodybuilding

"All thinking is a process of identification and integration. Man perceives a blob of color; by integrating the evidence of his sight and his touch, he learns to identify it as a solid object; he learns to identify the object as a table; he learns that the table is made of wood; he learns that the wood consists of cells, that the cells consist of molecules, that the molecules consist of atoms. All through this process, the work of his mind consists of answers to a single question: What is it? His means to establish the truth of his answers is logic, and logic rests on the axiom that existence exists. Logic is the art of non-contradictory identification. A contradiction cannot exist. An atom is itself, and so is the universe; neither can contradict its own identity; nor can a part contradict the whole. No concept man forms is valid unless he integrates it without contradiction into the total sum of his knowledge. To arrive at a contradiction is to confess an error in one's thinking; to maintain a contradiction is to abdicate one's mind and to evict oneself from the realm of reality."

John Galt, Ayn Rand
"Atlas Shrugged"

"Shake off all the fears of servile prejudices, under which weak minds are servilely crouched. Fix reason firmly in her seat, and call on her tribunal for every fact, every opinion. Question with boldness even the existence of a God; because, if there be one, he must more approve of the homage of reason, than that of blind-folded fear...Do not be frightened from this inquiry from any fear of its consequences. If it ends in the belief that there is no God, you will find incitements to virtue in the comfort and pleasantness you feel in its exercise..."

Thomas Jefferson, Third President of
The United States and Philosopher.

3

Theoretical Principles of Bodybuilding Exercise

> *"It is possible to fail in many ways...while to succeed is possible only in one way."*
>
> Aristotle

As I stated in the first chapter, confusion is the hallmark of today's bodybuilder. Through a brief examination of almost any commercial gym in the world, the rational observer witnesses that there is something decidedly wrong. In almost every case the observer witnesses that nearly every bodybuilder is frustrated with their results, or lack thereof—many working themselves into an emotional lather, expressing despondence and bewilderment for why they are not obtaining any manifestations of anything in the way of desired results, despite their religious devotion to exercise.

In the course of several months, maybe a year or two, many of the bodybuilders working out in a gym will simply give up, dejected—in many cases their self-esteem is left irreparably shaken. Without a doubt dear reader there is a problem in the world of bodybuilding today that is preventing progress. Countless bodybuilders set off on their bodybuilding programs with promiscuous abandon, perpetually confused and oblivious to the issue that not all, many or even two theories, including that of bodybuilding exercise, are of equal validity. However, as a result of their derisory growth from a few months (or years for some persistent bodybuilders) on a worthless routine or two most bodybuilders do not take it as evidence of the invalidity of the premise that all training theories are of equal value. Instead, intellectually superseded with confusion, they masochistically turn upon themselves out of fear and question their own physical-intellectual merit. A fear characterized by a preponderance of conflicting negative ideas percolating in greater and greater frequencies in their mind as they contemplate the possibility of some physical or psychological defect that prevents all the training routines they've used from allowing them to reach their goals. And this fear results in, if his premises are not corrected with rational re-examination, an epistemological upset for this bodybuilder, ensuing an anxious neurosis of self-damnation and a varying degree of hatred of the world that does not endow him so graciously and, seemingly, automatically as his idols.

For this reason the morally-intellectually shaken bodybuilder, the one who perseveres, turns back to the muscle magazines...unaware of anywhere else to turn to. They return, searching for the elusive answer via the biblical like commandments of their idols that continually tell him that only if their desire is great enough and if they persist and keep going to the gym for several hours everyday they will eventually succeed. And they are attracted to this quixotic mind-set, since everything they have heard in the culture suggests that if one is relentless and is a slave to his art, through sheer dint of merciless struggle, tireless sweat, he must succeed. After all, watching the bodybuilding videos of professional bodybuilders, such as Jay Cutler and Ronnie Colman, they see the top professionals spend, literally, all of their damn time training, eating, posing and sleeping.

Is it any wonder why bodybuilders today run around, buying vast numbers of bodybuilding magazines and books, workout DVDs and going to countless bodybuilding seminars…hoping, pleading, begging that one expert, anyone will someday, someway endow them with the esoteric knowledge that unlocks the secret of massive muscles.…Bodybuilders who eventually become full of contempt towards their sacrificial ideopraxist efforts, of which, are persuading no growth from their bodies.

But why are so many bodybuilders not attaining growth from their efforts, following the perfunctory ideologies of "They", this seemingly omniscient "They", the unbenounced inconclusive "They" that vary from supplement manufactures to the hodgepodge writers of the muscle magazines to semi-literate professionals? What is the arcane cause; what is the missing factor in their training efforts?

Without prolonging the issue, I will affirm that the realm of bodybuilding science is far more intellectually demanding that the average bodybuilder, and magazine writer recognizes. The missing factor of their unproductive training efforts is that they lack a conceptual grasp of what the *nature* of muscle is.

Nature sets the terms—In order to achieve a regular and deliberate effect from a particular entity you must first know its nature or identity, and then recognize identity's corollary: the law of causality. In order to deal with such a broad abstraction as the nature of muscular tissue, we must learn to think in principles. A principle being a fundamental primary or general truth, on which other truths depend. To quote Ayn Rand, "A principle is an abstraction which subsumes a great number of concretes. It is only by means of principles that one can set one's long-range goals and evaluate the concrete alternatives of any given moment. It is only principles that enable a man to plan his future and to achieve it."

The truth is the identification of some aspect of reality, and it is the intellectual absence and outright evasion of truth and, more fundamentally, principles that is the cause for the hindrance of productive exercise today and at all other times and issues where man has ignored reason for other means of gaining knowledge.

The definition of truth, however, has become distorted in our culture, anesthetized into illogical and mystical connotations, detached from reality in a numb dejection of subjectivity. But such is the dilemma of our age…the age of mankind's intellectual erosion. The field of bodybuilding science does not exist in a vacuum—do you honestly believe that bodybuilding would be exempt from this intellectual decay? No, I would presume that it would be one of the first to perpetrate stupidity, as virtually every so-called "specialist" or self-stylized expert in the field continues on with unchecked unchallenged premises of inappropriately applied, unrelated concepts and philosophies to exercise—lacking any scientific-objective foundation. It is not surprising that drowning in a cumulative, teratological ocean of inconclusive, contradictory answers the succumbing bodybuilder cries out with his last flicker of motivation to continue their bodybuilding efforts, "What is the truth and what judges whether it is true or not? Is it some omnipotent being or an overpaid crooked politician?"

As I stated in the previous chapter, reality is the ultimate arbiter of the truth. Reality dictates whether something is true or false. If you want to understand anything dealing within the realm of reality, the realm of the truth, you must adhere to reason. It is either/or, you cannot have it both ways. You have man's faculty to choose to accept and to conform to reality, to discover, understand and exploit the full potential of the world around you, including your body—as Francis Bacon said to eloquently, "*Nature, to be commanded must be obeyed.*" Or you can choose to remain blindly, fatally bewildered to life and the truth, festering in a state of an intellectual stillborn…. Except, whose reason do we judge by?

The answer is: you judge reality by a man's only means of survival—*your own* faculty of reason. No matter how vast or modest your knowledge, it is *your* mind that must acquire truth. Just as no one can breathe for you, eat for you, defecate for you; no one can think and understand for you. It is *your* mind that must deal with the content of *your* knowledge in order for you to be able to grasp the principles of reality. And there is and can only be one set of ultimately correct principles governing anything in reality, as there is only one reality, there can only be one, immutable theory of any aspect of it.

Despite the fact that it is true that every individual does posses a unique, one of a kind, personality and physical development that is impossible to replicate.

It is also true that anatomically and physiologically all human beings are essentially the same. Since we are dealing with the genus man, all of the physical attributes will be relative with all entities that have the common denominator of man. The only difference between individuals will be the measurement or degree of their human attributes (i.e. hair color, height, intelligence, skin color, etc.). This being true—birth defects and genetic abnormalities notwithstanding—a universal theory on any aspect of human physiology can and will be valid for everyone: a theory on nutritional needs, intellectual stimuli (audile, visual and physical contact), pain reception stimuli, perception (taste, smell, sight, touch and sound) and muscular growth stimuli (i.e. intense muscular contractions).

To assert that all theories are of equal value is to claim that a witch doctor in southern Africa, a practitioner with a success rate of virtually zero, is of equal value as our leading surgeons who practice Western medicine, with a success rate of nearly 100 percent. Such a claim is much more than ignorant; it is an outright and deliberate rejection of reason in favor of the inept, the utterly insane. To assert that Western technological advances have not advanced man beyond the primitive traditionalism of third world countries is to declare that you would be better off having your family live in the Amazon jungle where they have to fight everything from predator attack to disease caused by nothing more than a lack of a simple disinfectant!

* * *

In order to devise a correct theory on bodybuilding

exercise one must know the nature of the stimulus in order to define a valid theory of approach directed at enacting the most efficacious stimulus required for maximum desired results—along with an understanding of the counterproductive factors that need to be considered in order to avoid less than one-hundred percent productivity. And it is high intensity training that is the only universally demonstrable theory on human physiology that establishes how to develop muscular size and strength in the correct manner while keeping all of the potential negative factors of the stimulus in mind.

While high intensity training retains a hierarchy of logically interdependent principles and physiologic/psychological derivatives, the theory is founded upon three fundamental principles that are the three absolutes of any form of exercise: intensity, volume and frequency.

The Principle of Intensity

Dwindle down all factors of all means of obtaining any value and you will inevitable, in every case, come to one fundamental issue: *how hard did you have to work for it?* That is, what was the required intensity which was put forth to obtain it.

Muscle is quite the controversial tissue among today's many incompetent exercise physiologists. Sure, its composition and hormonal intricacies are rarely ignored or denied by even the most conceptually dim exercise physiologists, but the muscle's etiology, particularly in terms of muscle growth, digs into a whole history of criminal malpractice and self-arrested stupidity.

Today's current lot of exercise physiologists—with

very few rare exceptions—are the intellectual offspring of the same philosophical premises as professor Paul K. Feyerabend for whom held that, "The rationality of science does not really exist" and that "the special status and prestige of scientists are based on their own claims to objective truth [asserting that the sciences are not founded upon objective laws of the universe but on whim and wish of individuals who call themselves scientists]."

If you were to ask one of today's lucrative and renowned exercise physiologists how you would go about your bodybuilding or athletic training efforts you are, is almost every case, just wasting your time...or worse. Worse because you are endangering your wellbeing by following the Russian roulette of possible SWAG (scientific wild ass guesses). All you are told is to perform "Explosive lifting, like those Olympic weightlifters;" "Lift free weights to build muscular size, but utilize machines for muscular definition;" "Perform vibration training by standing on a platform and having the hell shook out of you;" "Train like the professionals and perform 12-20 sets per body parts six days a week;" "Train each body part from different angles;" ad infinitum—never why, just do it. What the hell is with all of the uncertainty?

In aeronautics, when you approach a pilot or an engineer and ask how do I get an airplane off the ground, you are usually given an answer that is a little more useful than, "Everyone is different...you have to find what works for you," or, "Explosives seem to put things in the air... why not try that," or, "Well...I see those hang gliders get in the air alright, why not push the damn thing off a cliff." ...Though there are many incompetent, supposed, "experts" in all fields, none seem to astound me more than those in the field of exercise. To paraphrase one of Mark Twain's famous remarks, "…In the first place God made idiots. This was for practice. Then he made exercise physiologists."

Today we lack a noteworthy pool of proper exercise physiologists—many of whom publish studies that never happened or publish conclusions that were gained from incorrectly analyzed data, sometimes by mistake…but mostly because of biasness. Individuals who ignore, even reticule, studies that are objectively demonstrable beyond any shadow of a doubt…but as Euripides once said, "Talk sense to a fool and he calls you foolish." Now don't get me wrong, there are some intelligent exercise physiologists out there (Martin Gibala and Mark Tarnopolsky of McMaster University are notable and Dr Ralph N. Carpinelli has recently caught my attention due to his intensive scrutiny of the scientific literature and his willingness to call out the myths and traditional misconceptions of his field), but such individuals are very few and far between.

But since we lack proper exercise physiologists, in general, we will take on the role of a proper one ourselves. How you ask? Well, instead of riffling through countless studies by other physiologists, looking for others who hold the same opinion or results as you so that you know that others will accept it, but making sure that you do not offend others so you make sure to state that their conclusions are correct too, like most exercise physiologists do, all that we will do is open our eyes.

Redirecting our attention from the contradictory clutter in the gym and the muscle/fitness magazines to a more generally understood subject, we (individuals who have ever seen two or more athletic competitions) are undeniably exposed to a practically self-evident difference between the long distance runner and the sprinter. On the issue of the results of their efforts, we are able to readily observe that most competitive sprinters possess a lower extremity muscularity to a degree that is parallel or superior to many natural bodybuilders, as against the long distance runners—an activity highlighted with many individuals that look as if they suffered in a Nazi concentration camp…and a continually growing number of such runners are actually suffered the same ultimate end. The problem at this point is deciphering the answer to muscle growth amid the characteristics of these two antitheses of resultants.

Many, supposed, experts in the field of exercise claim that it is the total amount of work performed that is the cause for greater degrees of muscle mass, but let's look at such a proposition seriously. A marathon runner covers *literally* hundreds of times more distance on foot than does the sprinter. A sprinter covers 100 to 200 yards in a race, while the marathon runner covers a minimum of 31,580 percent more distance—so, by way of the basic laws of physics, we see that the marathon runner performs 316.8 times as much *work* as the sprinter…so does that mean if you merely do less work you result in greater growth? Of course not! Such implications would imply that sitting at your computer would lead to the resultant of legs that would make Tom Platz look like an individual befallen with a muscle wasting disease. In these two opposing activities, literally almost all factors involved are *identical*—the sum of caloric energy utilized to perform a given amount of work is the same, whether you jog or all-out sprint 200 yards, it makes no slightest difference in the amount of energy used; the biomechanical movements of the body are also almost identical in both activities.

The factor in your efforts that is directly responsible for the stimulation of muscle growth is not the *quantity* of effort but the *quality* or *intensity* of effort. And it has been shown, indisputably (though when has that ever stopped people from blindly arguing a subject that is irrefutable—e.g. The Flat Earth Society, a group of people who believe that the world is flat), that the most important requirement for stimulating an increase in muscular size and strength is the imposition of a high intensity muscular contraction.[1] A longer duration is not important in this equation and does not yield further muscle growth, as was shown by Roux-Lange. Roux-Lange demonstrated that only when a muscle contracts with its greatest power by overcoming a greater resistance in a unit of time would it hypertrophy. Furthermore, Lange discovered that if a muscle were made to perform work for merely a longer period of time with the same resistance as before, the muscle would not increase in size.[2]

What's more, a high intensity muscular contraction actually prevents you from performing a long duration and large number of such contractions. Try this experiment if you don't believe me. Tomorrow, take a 30-mile walk and make a mental note of your experiences…whether you liked the sound of the birds chirping as you walk by or how you enjoyed a friendly mutual wave from your old school mate, etc. Now the very next day, attempt to reach that very same 30-mile displacement again, but!

This time, run at full tilt from square one to the finish (*and I mean run, as fast as you can, non-stop!*). Mentally note your experiences during that run….Almost certainly you'll notice little, if anything, besides finding yourself facedown in a pool of your own saliva, in a life and death struggle to get any amount of air into your lungs after one mile—if that.

Though this fact is simple and undeniable, it runs in direct opposition to what most of the coaches, personal trainers and gym teachers out there believe and inculcate their students with—the fact that *intensity and duration exist in an inverse ratio to one another*, as Mike Mentzer stated, "You can train hard or you can train long, but you can't do both." And once the duration begins to increase, the intensity of that activity follows suit with a proportionate decrease—as it must for the reason that you only possess a finite reserve of readily available energy to draw upon. Moreover, it is a practically self-evident fact that when most of that finite reserve is devoted towards length of activity instead of intensity the outcome is less than positive in terms of muscle growth…but since this simple, nearly omnipresent fact is ignored, hundreds of millions of man-hours of training and tens of billions of foot-pounds of effort are wasted annually to programs that result in a level of progress in 3 years that could have, should have, been attained in 3 months or less.

* * *

Understand that a muscular contraction performed at a very high degree of intensity is all that is physiologically required in order to *stimulate* muscular growth. The keyword in the matter of your workout is that, it stimulates muscle growth; the workout itself does not produce muscular growth, but *purely,* stimulates a potential of growth. The performance of a high intensity muscular contraction is universal in its *potential* to induce increases in both muscular size and strength to a degree that, if the body is left undisturbed, almost defies belief. But now the intelligent reader asks, why and how?

In 1865, Claude Bernard published his theory of an organism's physiological tendency to maintain a state of equilibrium, metabolically within a cell and an organism. Walter B. Cannon, the famous Harvard physiologist, subsequently called this power to maintain constancy in living beings *Homeostasis.* This discovery by Claude Bernard is very important in the explanation of the physiologic requirement of high intensity muscular work, as we will see.

The human body has an extraordinary ability to remain in a very narrow margin of a preferred internal environment: body temperature, acidity, acquiring nutritional needs, etc. The human body's ability to remain in a homeostatic state is so persevering that, for instance, its internal temperature can stay at its vitally important warmth of 98.2°F in sub-zero climates with little clothing for hours. The body is an extremely stubborn and immensely sophisticated survival organism. For that reason, you must realize that if you are demanding the human body to change internally and risk compromising its ability to survive famine and drought you are going to have to force it to do so! And the only way to create an extraordinarily biologically demanding and metabolically expensive growth is by the imposition of a significant threat to your system.

The body has within it, defense mechanisms situated to defend itself from aggressive stresses, allowing the individual a chance to survive and then adapt—but they will only be activated if absolutely required.

There exists a part of your brain that continuously, automatically monitors both your current activity and the metabolic requirements for the performance of these activities. In the process of this continual monitoring, when the brain identifies that the body has encountered a stress that pushes its current physical ability to the limit (the imposition of a high intensity muscular contraction) there is an unconscious, vital, decision made: the body, based on previous experiences, identifies that it requires a change toward a physical state that is more up to the task of the demands of this type and degree of stress.

When you are forcing your body to work near the absolutely limit of its current ability, the body will then decide that it needs to grow stronger. And if you do nothing to prevent your body's internal processes of adaptation, your body will grow stronger and consequently bigger, along with the other requisite physiologic structural adaptations that make such an increase in strength tolerable: increased muscular endurance; increased cardiovascular ability; increased functional and structural strength of your bones, tendons, ligaments, heart and other organs.

When in pursuit of an increase of muscular size and strength your goal is to literally threaten the body with a high intensity stressor that the body perceives as a life and death struggle—i.e. exercise performed with high intensity tells your body (as it perceives it) that it has two choices: grow stronger or die. But intensity is a confusing term, due to the fact that there are so many "experts" proclaiming different definitions...and what exactly is "high" intensity?

The most accurate way to correctly define intensity is, *intensity is the percentage of momentary ability.* What high intensity can be defined as is *the maximum percentage of possible momentary muscular effort capable of being exerted.* Meaning that, it is only that last, seemingly impossible, repetition of a set carried to a point of momentary muscular failure, where an individual is forced to exert every ounce of his momentary strength that is of true high intensity.

As you near the end of the set, as the momentary level of strength of the muscles being utilized continues to fall as a result of accumulating fatigue, the last few repetitions will feel considerably harder than the preceding, because, by that point, the remaining strength that your muscles are capable of generating is so low that just about all of your strength is required to just prevent the weight from coming down—let alone lifting it.

If you continue to the point were you fail, where you are literally not strong enough to perform another repetition with proper form, no matter how hard you try, then only one repetition in the entire set actually involved high intensity: the last repetition. Thus, "high intensity" training is performing an exercise to the point of momentary muscular failure by means of generating the highest possible intensity or force you are capable of on the last, hardest, repetition of the exercise.

As a homeostatic organism, the human body makes it its top priority to resist change. It requires, by its *nature*, a staggeringly immense degree of persuasion in order for it to deem it necessary to change. It is in that last repetition of a set carried to the point momentary muscular failure, where you are trying to move the weight as hard as possible, where you are gritting your teeth, shaking all over and are unable to move it, even slightly, that is particularly special. All of the preceding repetitions were ineffective in activating the growth mechanism of the body, as they were not physiologically *threatening* enough. (And ending a set just because some arbitrary prescription of repetitions is reached will do absolutely nothing to stimulate muscle growth—your muscles are able to tolerate it.) It is only by attempting those last one or two repetitions that you will be able to dip into what is called your reserve ability—this reserve ability seems to be an evolutionarily necessary capacity, required for a last-ditch effort to flee or kill one of mankind's early predators.

With the performance of a high intensity workout, we are not acting in the direction of a casual social activity, but *a life-threatening struggle against death!* All of the repetitions before the last seemingly impossible one were only preparatory. It is during that last one or two repetitions that your body undergoes an extraordinary metabolic change. Digging into this reserve ability tells your body that it must become stronger for the sake of making sure that the next time it meets this type of foe (the weights in our case) it will have some reserve ability left to insure survival.

Reaching that last nearly impossible repetition, it is at that moment that you notice that you do not feel the same as you did when you started the exercise, or even the few prior repetitions. Not just in the muscles that were exercised, but systemically: your breathing is very rapid, your pulse is high and a general sense of fatigue, even nausea, is experienced. You experience the fact that you have created a deficit in your body and, consequently, you have become temporarily weaker...weaker to such a degree that you are usually momentarily incapable of lifting the afflicted limb itself immediately after finishing the set. And it is with that one, final, maximal repetition that you have effectively sent your ultimatum to your body—grow or die!

Though it may sound like I am belaboring the issue, I can assure you that, if anything, I am leaving far too much out. Repetition is the paramount method to learn anything, and since most have been, and are currently being, inculcated relentlessly by half-truths and whole lies on the matter of what stimulates muscles to grow, mentioning the truth once usually will not penetrate the wall of fallacy erected in many individuals' minds.

* * *

It is that last rep that sets in motion the *growth mechanism* of the body. Now understand that I am not speaking metaphorically when I speak of a growth mechanism; the body does in fact possess a growth mechanism that is tied into the central nervous system. Consequently, since the central nervous system does not just supply a particular muscle, but the entire body, it begins a general, systemic chain reaction of metabolic adaptations throughout the entire body.

This mechanism I speak of is actually an internal defense mechanism of the body used to maintain a homeostatic state. As aforementioned, the body was already acknowledged to endure in maintaining a state of internal equilibrium by Claude Bernard. However, the manner in which the body defends itself against stress was not understood until it was theoretically established and clearly defined by Dr. Hans Selye with his General Adaptation Syndrome (G.A.S.).

While we view such things as the deepening of a suntan or the buildup of muscular mass as purely cosmetic, the body did not have such in mind. The compensatory buildup of muscular mass is a physiologic defense mechanism used to protect the body from the physiologic threat of exhausting, intense muscular stress. The body truly despises the process of increasing its level of muscular size beyond the essential, as a former cohort of Mike Mentzer once said in response to the statement that man was an instinctual creature, "If man were to follow his instincts he would defecate or urinate on a barbell—he certainly would not lift it!"

The Principle of Volume

*"Measure not the work until the day's out
and the labor done."*
Elizabeth Barrett Browning

Intensity is the first and foremost requisite of productive bodybuilding exercise. Though, once the fundamental principle of intensity is grasped we still do not possess the necessary foundation to define a correct theory of bodybuilding exercise. The principle of intensity has a corollary that, once the muscle is made to perform the proper level of intensity, must be taken into the equation if the stimulation induced by the workout's intensity is to be actualized: the volume of the workout.

The General Adaptation Syndrome, Dr. Selye explains, states that the body reacts to stress in three distinct physiologic stages. Stage one is the general alarm stage, stage two is the stage of resistance, and stage three is the stage of exhaustion. In demonstrating the body's physiologic reaction to stress, I will use the generally understood concept of ultra violet radiation exposure for the purpose of tanning alongside the effects of exercise for the purpose of muscle growth.

The General Alarm Stage: The first stage of general alarm is initiated with the first exposure to an intense dosage of ultra violet radiation, which initially causes redness to appear and a slight inflammation to occur as the sun's radiation damages the sensitive membranes of the epidermis. With intense exercise there is an awareness of feeling fatigued that is accompanied with a muscular state of being temporarily weaker. After exposure to stress has been recognized by the body it will react upon this stimulus with the second stage—the stage of resistance.

The Stage of Resistance: In the case of ultra violet radiation exposure, when the body is left alone to compensate for the biochemical resources the stress consumed and given additional time to adapt by overcompensating, the body will start to produce melanin to combat and acclimatize itself to the stress, producing a tan. In the case of exercise, after allowing time for the body to recuperate and then to adapt to the toll of intense exercise, it will respond with a compensatory buildup of muscular tissue.

So while we adapt and respond to stress in proportion to its intensity, we also use up proportionate reserves of adaptation energy. In other words, the greater the intensity the more adaptation energy we use up. So therefore, the more sets we perform the greater the deficit of our adaptive energy reserves.

While Dr. Selye never proved it climactically, he believed that we possess local reserves of adaptation energy that are used up initially as we adapt to stress. This draining of the local reserves is what leads us to stop a bodybuilding workout at a certain point. Only if we were to go pass the point where our bodies are able to adapt or even recover and were to continue on with exposure to the stress would we enter the final stage—the stage of exhaustion.

The Stage of Exhaustion: In this stage, when we are dealing with ultra violate radiation, continuing exposure without time to merely compensate for the drain the stress has taken from the body, we will begin to develop a sunburn. Then, if continued further, we will begin to develop blisters as the tissues of the body begin to deteriorate and, if carry to such extremes, we will eventually die. Exercise carried out in such a fashion soon leads to a complete cessation in progress and then an eventual loss of muscle tissue followed by, if carried to extremes, death.

Dr. Selye contended that there is a local or superficial adaptation energy reserve that is immediately available upon demand. However, Dr. Selye further contended that there is a deep adaptation energy that is stored away, safely, as a last resort reserve. This reserve is different from the reserve ability that we are trying to tap with high intensity exercise…this one is a sort of chemical reserve. A temporary demand like a high intensity workout is reversible, but the exhaustion of our reserves of deep adaptation energy is not reversible. This deep adaptation energy could be histological components of heart, lung, bone, and nervous tissues. When these deep reserves are depleted in normal life, the result is senility and, finally, death.

* * *

Muscle growth is our body's defensive mechanism to increase its physiologic margins of stress tolerance. Your goal as an intelligent and rational bodybuilder is to enact the alarm stage with the imposition of the appropriate stress or intensity. Then, with the goal of a compensatory increase in muscular size and strength kept well in mind, allow the defensive mechanisms of the body to recover the superficial adaptive energy and biochemical resources, repair microscopic muscular tears and allow cellular inflammation to subside that the workout induced. Followed by allowing the body enough time to overcompensate with a surplus of muscle tissue.

Yet, despite this imperative and practically self-evident necessity, chronic arbitrary dogma has bewildered the field of bodybuilding ever since its conception. Systematically though, all of the routines and training systems, ranging from Bob Hoffman to Joe Weider to Arthur Jones to Charles Poliquin, end at the one fundamental question: how many sets should one perform?

It is truly distressing how the cardinal application of logic in science today as a whole, bodybuilding science notwithstanding, is seldom used. Though this can only be anticipated, seeing that the irrationalities of the Kantian philosophy that have weeded in since the turn of 19th century. A philosophy advocating such subjective notions as absolutes do not exist, reality is not real and man is an impotent being incapable of gaining knowledge, all of which are proliferating in the moral province of truth and divert it from reality.

The *Reductio ad absurdum* of today's experts, the intellectually bereft, is the "more is better" philosophy that is seen as critically significant in the economic, emotional and social trades: more money is better than less, more happiness is better than less, more friends are better than less, so why not more exercise. It only seems "self-evident" that more exercise is better than less right? Wrong! In fact, nothing is self-evident except the matter provided by the senses. Understanding the fundamental requirements of a correct approach to economics, psychology, politics and bodybuilding exercise goes beyond the self-evident into the highly abstract that are not directly perceivable. The ignorance of the more is better reasoning is, as Mike Mentzer repetitively retorted, trying to apply the childish-like logic that more jellybeans are better than less, so theorizing that the same must apply to exercise— more exercise must be better than less. However, you soon come to realize that this notion is erroneous as at a certain point eating jellybeans you become sick! You realize that eating more jellybeans has only made you fat, a negative consequence, and the same ultimate result of a negative applies for exercise as well. Although the notion of "more is better" is attractive in its simplicity, it simply does not work.

Stimulus>>>Organism>>>Response

The above equation is a simple theoretical formula used in pharmaceuticals for testing drugs. The application of such formula is equally valid for high intensity training, as we are dealing with the same thing: a drug or better described as a stimulus that enacts a physiologic/ metabolic response from the body being subjected to it. So in order to demonstrate the significance of this formula's application, let us create a hypothetical situation with two individual human subjects and substitute the stimulus in this equation with two different stimuli: weight training and a standard general anesthetic. The organisms in this situation are the bodies of these two individuals and the response is their body's reaction to their respective stimuli.

For the sake of this hypothetical situation, we will first administer a low amount of training intensity and an average amount of volume to one individual and a low administration of the general anesthetic to the other. What is the response of the organisms: note, if anything, the individuals will respond with little physiologic/ biochemical change...leaving one with absolutely no growth stimulated and the other running out of the surgical suite before the surgeon begins the incision. Now if we were to administer the precise requisite dosage of general anesthetic and of weight training volume and intensity to elicit the desired results what is the response of the organisms: in one, we have successfully imposed a state of anesthesia and stimulated large muscular tissue growth potential in the other without compromising either subject's safety and health.

However, if we were to continue to administer

the anesthetic and the training stimuli volume, we will produce a quiet different response from the organisms. We find that, with continual administration of the general anesthetic, the one subject responds by going into a coma and/or dies and in the other individual there is no gain and eventually a loss of tissue—not just skeletal muscular tissue—and even death in extremely persistent cases with exercise. This weight lifting over-dosage effect was acutely demonstrated with the near death of former Mr. America Steve Michalik. Steve advocated the performance of extremely high volume in weight training and insisted on training each body part with 75 to 100 sets a workout! Steve practiced what he preached and, because of which, being true to his motto, "Train beyond the pain...and death is your only release", he nearly died.

You must realize that proper and intelligent high intensity training is not the simplistic act of performing more or less than everyone else, but performing only the *required* amount needed in order to induce the desired physiologic response. And, after doing so, if the body is allowed to recuperate and its defense mechanisms are left undisturbed to adapt, the body will react with the desired physiologic change. But how many sets are precisely required in proper high intense training? Is it the performance of four exercises, 3 sets each of 10 repetitions as recommended by one professional or is it three exercises, 4 sets of 12 repetitions recommended by another or the classic 12-20 sets recommended by Joe Weider and Arnold Schwarzenegger?

So we now come full circle. How many sets are required in order to stimulate maximum muscle growth? Well, how many bullets are required to kill you? How many sperm were needed to stimulate growth of your mother's ovum into a fully-fashioned human being, i.e. you? How many flicks of a light switch are required to turn on a light? How many sets are required by muscle's nature in order to stimulate optimum and spectacular gains in muscular size and strength without compromising the body's biochemical resources? One. One is all that is required by the nature of these entities to achieve these respective ends.

Some individuals reading this will state, "Well what if you miss with a bullet, possess defective sperm and the light bulb is broken?" To these smart-aleck individuals I would like to reiterate the point that we are being logically precise: straight through the eyes, cell division of the ovum into a zygote, hitting the light switch with a working light bulb and performing one set to momentary muscular failure. Or as I said to my friend Brandon Robitaille when reiterating the point of only performing the least amount of exercise required, "There are thousands of exercises that you can perform and an equally staggering number of sets possible… just like there are thousands of ways to kill yourself. But if you get it right the first time you don't have to do it again!" The contemplation of this dramatic fact is not surprisingly seen as controversial. How can it only be one?

Well, why not? If you properly build a house, how many times must you build it before it is built? How many compound factures do you need in order to say that your arm is broken? If you cannot accept or are just not comfortable with the introduction to this valid concept requiring only one set, you can alter the standard of notation and, instead of seeing it as only one set, imagine it as 100 or even 100,000 units of intensity.

Instead of obsessing over the numerical unit of one let us focus on the *nature* of one set of high intensity exercise carried to failure, which can be flawlessly analogized to hitting a stick of dynamite with a hammer. *One* precise and intense hit is all that is required, but it is capable of, and it will achieve, an enormous amount of productivity.

The only precondition of that one set, that is capable of literally almost unimaginable results, is that *it must be intense*. Nothing in life is free, as the old adage goes "There is no such thing as a free meal", and this is true, as you cannot gain *anything* without effort being involved. Anyone who would tell you otherwise is either a crook who is just trying to sell you some worthless, even dangerous, piece of junk while fronting a bullshit smile(such things as the sauna belt and vibrating platforms come to mind) or simply stupid—frequently both. There is no such thing as an "easy" form of *productive* exercise…there is, however, a very quick and productive form of exercise, but in no way is it close to being easy. If that one set is going to do anything you will have to give it everything you got, and this is to be taken literally.

You will feel an accumulating pain, not indicative of injury or a precursor to any harm, but it will be an intensifying burning and a discomforting numbing ache that will turn you off immediately. It will make you want to quite then and there if you are not psychologically prepared, as every second beyond the comfort threshold the numbing ache unceasingly builds. Nevertheless, you can't give up, not if you want to grow. Anything less than everything that you can give is, in almost every case, just a waste of time, and results in an outcome that is generally less pleasurable than the act of overloading your muscles, i.e. no positive results.... Chew on that the next time you are nearing the final reps of a set...and know this, if you are intent on achieving stronger and larger muscles, it's all or nothing! Anything less is mere guesswork in the productivity of your efforts, anymore is virtually impossible...it leaves no room for error...taken to failure you can be damn sure that that set of intense exercise crossed any threshold required for your body to deem growth indispensable.

Those of you who will still not deem that this valid training theory is justifiable or even possible need only look around to see the error in your premise. Man has technologically progressed unfathomably in the last 200 years and has evolved conceptually at the same pace. Simply look around you, look at the machines we have now, look at the performance of our Olympic athletes, and look at the medical sciences, astronautics, the internet, cell phones, computers, TV, and food! Technologically, we have become a completely new class of being, as we have become more efficacious by understanding the identity of reality and its laws of causality.

You say the idea of training for 2 to 5 minutes and obtaining spectacular results is impossible. The same impossibility was declared for space exploration—Apollo was the perfect name for man's break into the sunlight and his heroic recognition of truth.

Once man begins to understand the nature of an entity it is only a matter of time before he will become more economically efficient and produce the greatest with the least amount of resources required to express the entity's inherent potential. You question the potential of man's mind? I would advise you to gaze up into the clear night's sky. That is what man is capable of achieving.

The Principle of Frequency

"Being one of the crowd—particularly when the crowd doesn't know what it's doing—shouldn't be something any rational individual would want to be a part of"

John Little

When applying the appropriate knowledge to any subject in reality, the sought after resultant of your efforts should be nothing short of spectacular—this being equally true for bodybuilding as well.

Correct bodybuilding exercise has three primary principles that are equally vital and indivisible in the pursuit of the greatest muscular size and strength gains possible. They are intensity, volume and frequency. Since we have already discussed the principles of intensity and volume let us now consider the final principle of frequency.

If you were to glance through a current muscle magazine you would observe, besides its overwhelming ostentatious push of supplements, exercise equipment and the like, that all of the professional bodybuilders recommend exercising 4 to 6 days a week, one to even four times a day. It would seem in light of this glistening bible of chiseled bodies and scantily clothed women that exercise performed more often is superior to less—and never is it asked or explained why, only hollowed with a logicless resonance of, "why not?"

The most widespread fallacy (one of countless others) of nearly all bodybuilders, sports/strength coaches, personal trainers, physiotherapists and exercise scientists (to name a few) is that of an integration of a long referred to, baseless, floating abstraction with exercise: that "more" equates to "better." But if exercise, as espoused by the Pros, our self-asserted experts, is a good thing because it "produces" muscle growth, as we are told, why not produce further growth by training more often. To take their ideology's equivocal axiom seriously, if "more is better" is the correct theory of bodybuilding exercise, why would you only train 6 days a week, four times a day for an hour? Such only seems moronic when you can take the next four months off from work, workout everyday for 20 hours and in no time you would seize the intense muscularity and thickness of Dorian Yates. You should now realize how absurd the notion that more is better is when one attempts to apply it to bodybuilding exercise.

Frequency or, more technically precise, recovery time must, and I am above all serious about this point, it must be as equally valued as much as the workout itself. If your goal is unprecedented gains in muscular size and strength you must understand the importance of recovery in the logically interdependent hierarchy of your bodybuilding program. It is 50-50 with neither of the two elements being of greater value than the other is—as without the workout, there is no incentive for growth and without recovery time, there is no instance of the allotted time required for the body to produce a compensatory build-up of muscle mass.

Returning to the routines of the professional bodybuilders, we come to an interesting situation…there are only one or three days a week permitted for recovery…a piss poor amount of time allotted for growth, seeing that your muscles do not recover and grow in the gym. However, immediately upon being told this statement, the intellectually staunched bodybuilder retorts, ignorant of the slew of tremendous recovery enhancing properties huge quantities of steroids and growth hormone possess, that their adorned muscled heroes train different body parts on different days as to allow those muscles that are not being directly used time to recover.

However, contrary to what a good number of bodybuilders believe, your muscles do not function completely independently from one another and they do not draw upon biochemical resources solely from their own reserve of glycogen and other substrates stored within them. You possess only one body, one enclosed environment with every change of one component of it influencing the whole to some degree. An attempt to recover a muscle simply by not using it in the proceeding workout the next day or later that same day is either pure neophytic ignorance or just unadulterated stupidity (I myself was once the latter of the two).

The performance of an exercise, no matter what that exercise may be—be it a squat, a cable crossover, a lying triceps extension, or even a preacher curl—enacts a *systemic* drain upon the entire body's reserve of biochemical resources. The severity of the drain you make of these resources must be realized as the determinate of how much of your body's *limited* adaptation energy will have to be diverted towards refilling this debt, as whatever sum of energy left after that serves the body in adapting to the workout by increasing its stress tolerance. Furthermore, just like everything else in the universe—including the universe itself—the body only has a *limited* reserve of such resources to draw upon.

And just like any other drain of a resource, it requires time to restore the sum depleted. Recall earlier I mentioned that the workout itself does not produce muscular growth but merely stimulates it. In order to acquire the growth potential you stimulated in the workout you must allow the body to recovery the debt that the workout accumulated and then, and only then, allow the body itself to overcompensate in the form of a muscle size and strength increase. The topic of central concern at this point is how frequently do you need to train in order to gain muscle at an unimpeded rate?

* * *

Someone once said that, "We learn, when we learn, only from experience; and then only from our mistakes; our successes merely serve to reinforce our superstitions." And, while this is not true in absolute terms, I have yet to see an one example to prove that merely inculcating someone with theory and beliefs is better than having them experience the matter at hand themselves, attempt to learn from the mistakes that they make—and there will usually be many—and then allowing them to form an opinion of the matter from their attempts to correct their mistakes. However, if you were to look at the educational systems of both the United States and Canada you would see that this is not the way these governments believe that schools should conduct their efforts.

One thing that I have noticed is that we learn, if we do at all, primarily from our most serious mistakes—that includes mankind's seemingly endless history of mistakes; and our most pernicious mistake that our countries are making is the time-honored act of ignoring the past. History class used to be the most important class in your education—so important in fact that failing it would automatically hold you back a year…why? Because prior to the "progressive educational" ethos of John Dewey, before the educational system became fubar, as they say in the military, it was recognized that the most important class for a child's development is the study of history, because history class is nothing but a long list of mistakes people made and a short list of individuals who were able to learn from them and take a step forward towards where we are now…but why was this so important? Well when you are able to learn why things like the dark ages, mass ritualistic killings, the rise of Nazism and Communism, and many such things took place, you become a little more prone to avoid the same mistakes and spare yourself the grief of learning from those kinds of mistakes the hard way.

But the educational system today is a pragmatic election of one haphazard idea after another. History classes today, among all other courses, have been so violently twisted and manipulated to fit the "politically correct" majority consensus that to call it anything less than a merciless killing of mankind's intellectual giants and a heroic applause for the murderous actions of the Attila's and Nero's of history is nothing short of vile. But this is what the majority desire and want, it is what they believe is best…sure, but as someone once said…"Just where and when has it ever been demonstrated that the majority are right about anything?"

A result of the "teachings" in classrooms today is that most kids and teenagers have become ignorant and lazy. When they are having difficulty in a course, instead of making an effort to further assist the student or holding them back for the benefit of having a chance to fully grasp the subject, they are usually just pushed through to the next grade. I have heard the whining and complaining of students bewailing because they have two or three pages to read over the weekend, that they have to study for a test, that their exams are "too hard"...the results? Well the school boards cave-in and dumb down the curriculum, remove the harder material, reduce, or even eliminate homework.

What does this have to do with bodybuilding? A whole lot actually. Bodybuilding is a discipline that requires meticulous thought and reflection. Above all, the results of our bodybuilding efforts are an either/or matter of focus and personal struggle that is not subject to the whim of "It is too hard...I want it now...but I don't want to work for it." The actual enormous benefit of proper strength training exercise is lost when the individual that has everything to gain from it does not because it is uncomfortable, tiring, difficult, etc. And this laziness has resulted in a tremendous downfall of bodybuilding interest at the level of average individuals.

A trait that is far too common among the genetically gifted individuals of the bodybuilding world is the misinterpretation of obtaining a progressive, desirable, result—a result due not to their actions but a result of their superhuman genetic disposition—and then emboldening it in their mind that the method that they used is the one

"true" answer to this issue of building bigger muscles...
but more often than not, it is usually wrong.

The genetic freaks (as is the term of endearment in
bodybuilding lingo for genetically gifted individuals)
have the natural potential to grow to beyond average
degrees of muscularity and strength *in spite* of their
efforts...many such rare individuals develop beyond the
average physical state with absolutely nothing in the way
of exercise. The difficulty with identifying the needed
frequency between workouts today is that the majority
of individuals that pickup an interest in bodybuilding
look to the professionals due to the mistake of equating
muscular size with intelligence...which of coarse is not
to say that professional bodybuilders are dumb, I would
say that many bodybuilders are far brighter than most
scientists, but most do not even have the slightest clue as
to the simple requirements of proper exercise.

(And to try to explain to them that their training
is holding them back or actually preventing them from
gaining any more muscle when they have invested
countless hours training in that manner is only an exercise
in futility. It takes an enormous amount of courage to
admit a personal mistake and then only an individual of
true intelligence and honesty will actually be able to learn
from it—and finding such an individual will have you
very hard-pressed.)

Failure tells you that something is wrong...but when
most people have gained even a negligible degree of
success—unless they are an individual who is in an ever-
active pursuit of the truth and are not dissuaded by the
possibility of finding errors in their own judgment—they
will usually become resistant to change, even if they later

discover that their method is flawed...why? Fear...the fear of being wrong and having people know it. And fear can make people do some very stupid things.

The problem with the routines that are espoused by the physique elite is that the individuals that actually gain on them are blind to the error in their actions. A semi-positive result, as incremental as it is, is usually the pitfall of discovering the truth for most people, even more so today with the intellectual state of most people. Since laziness is easy, most people confine their intellectual temperament to the maxim of, "If it worked for someone else, why change it? He built 20 inch arms; he must know what he is doing." Sure. The current economic collapse that we are experiencing today (2008/2009) is fundamentally the very same factor for the lack of progress in the efforts of the majority of bodybuilders: individuals are not questioning the actions and edicts of their peers and the experts.

Nonetheless, to be subdued by the fact that some individual progressed on an absurd four hour long routine, performed six to seven times a week, which would kill an adult gorilla, not questioning his routines' correctness on the basis that that particular individual built a 20 inch arm, and then submissively following his program because of which, will only have you only wasting countless hours in heartache. Such an individual did not burn the candle at both ends for months or years to formulate such a routine, he is a rare individual that could probably just look at a barbell and he would grow.

But instead of a reasoned approach that he sought for, one that was universally applicable and the most productive manner for him to achieve his goals, he just started lifting weights and discovered that he could grow quickly. Then he found that, even when he trained twice as long he was still able to grow more than the other individuals training in the gym were. Now, correlating his growth with exercise, he decided that since some exercise was giving him results and twice as much exercise was still giving him better results than everyone else was getting around him, more must be better. And since he was progressing appreciably on his routine, he decides that he must share his revolutionary, earth-shaking knowledge with the rest of the individuals in the gym… because if it worked for him, it will work for everyone if they training forever and a day, just like him….Is it any wonder that, in all probability, more than 70 percent of individuals that take up bodybuilding quit within a year after following the advice of the professionals. But, really, what did you expect from listening to the advice of the mystics of muscle?

The greatest obstacle to progress in science is the illusion of knowledge…the illusion that you already know what is going on when you don't even have the slightest clue. And I have been prevented from making further progress more times than I care to image, all because a previous concept that I held to be true at the time was false, but I believed it to be true as it yielded a result.

When an individual finds that they have gained a degree of success from their efforts, they will usually fight to the death, crying out that their method was the best manner to get where they are now, even when confronted with the simple facts of reality that prove otherwise…but such are the ethos of fear.

Now most, if not all, people who look at the results

produced by professional bodybuilders will deem such as being good…but good is a relative term. Good compared to what? Good compared to the growth of a bedridden individual with a muscle wasting disease—sure. But comparing the *end* results produced by one individual to another is worthless for the purpose of assessing the effectiveness of their training. You must judge things in context; you cannot meaningfully evaluate something without having a clear understanding of the relationship between the purported benefits and their actual costs. As someone once said…"First look at the results; but even then you must view them in context for any real understanding."

You say that it took someone only fifteen years to build fifty pounds of muscle…if so, I can honestly say that their results are not good…pathetic may still be too weak of a word to appraise such results. Don't get me wrong, the potential of producing a muscular surplus of fifty pounds is significant by any standard…but the amount of time put forth in exchange for that rate of growth over a fifteen year period is so far in the way of excess that I can assure you that at least ninety percent of that time and effort in the gym was wasted, almost certainly, it only served to hold them back from faster, or even better, gains.

But who am I to question their actions? How in the hell do I assert that they are wrong and I am right when I do not hold a bodybuilding championship title or a PhD? Well it does not matter who is wrong and who is right; all that matter is *what is correct*. I—the theory of high intensity bodybuilding exercise, from Arthur Jones to SuperSlow to Max Contraction to Heavy Duty—have demonstrable evidence of the fact that intense, brief and infrequent exercise is not only, without a lingering doubt, the only universal method of increasing muscular size and strength but also the most productive. Examples of such individuals that have benefited to a degree that they were never able to achieve before high intensity training run into the hundreds of thousands or more in the United States alone, but more recognizable names would be Dorian Yates, David Paul of the famous Barbarian brothers, Mike and Ray Mentzer, Aaron Baker, Casey Viator, David Mastorakis, Markus Reinhardt and John Heart (to name a few).

Instead of confining your intellectual range to the idiotic method of assessing something's worth by who said it, focus solely on *what* they said—*substance* is infinitely more important than *source*. Far too many people have been lead down the primrose path of false promises, only to later find themselves on the wrong end of a gun or a machete because they were judging people by name instead of by what they were actually saying and doing.

Likewise, far too many geniuses from times long pass to today are ignored and scrutinized all because they did not have a "name" or a position in the scientific/social community, usually due to the fact that they presented something new, something theoretically radical—resulting in scientific revolutions that would have brought us into a new era of technological advancement, cures for innumerable diseases that kill millions and the mass production of astounding products that would make life today far better, all becoming lost because "the powers that be" disagreed, seeing as these ideas were new, contrary to the accepted, would put the lie to the ideas of the leading experts.... Individuals such as Nikola Tesla were never given their due credit…but of coarse your AC current, radio, hydroelectric dams, radar, florescent lights, loud speakers and MRI/ X-ray machines (to name some of his brilliant inventions) would have all been developed by the scientific community and the government without him, right? Well if they didn't spend most of their time attacking his ideas, destroying his image and trying to steal his inventions, I guess they could have found some time to invent something of value…but I highly doubt that.

* * *

Returning to the initial point: how often should you be training? Well that is a very difficult question to answer—just who is asking. I have mentioned that there exist specific fundamental characteristics that all human beings share—resulting in my earlier statement that everyone, physiologically and anatomically, are essentially the same. Although such is true, everyone is different…different by way of measurement in their human characteristics. The issue of frequency is the matter of, are you training infrequently enough for your body's recovery ability to compensate for the exhaustive effects of the workout. The subject of recovery ability though—which I will cover in detail in the next chapter—has caused the whole of bodybuilding exercise science to be swoon by rare individuals with the idiosyncratic genetic ability to recover from nonsensically long and frequent workouts—individuals that ensure you that your quixotic fantasy of possessing 20 inch arms and a 60 inch chest is within your grasp, but only if you are willing to devote your life to the gym.

The issue of recovery needs is dependent on the intensity and volume of work that is performed. If you are an average forty-year-old male who has not trained or done any demanding physical activity for a period of several years, training to failure with six or seven exercises two times a week will be realistically assured to allow you adequate recovery time—you are literally too weak at that point to overwhelm your recovery ability on a twice a week frequency. Nevertheless, due to the nature of this type of work (high intensity exercise) a frequency of twice a week with six or seven exercises will soon become inadequate for the recovery needs of a much stronger and larger muscle—a fourteen inch arm contracting maximally does not produce the same demands on the body as that same arm two inches larger. For the general population a frequency of once every five to seven days is optimal, but not permanent—yes, some individuals will have the rare genetic ability to train three times a week and yield slightly faster results in a month's time, but these individuals too would do better to train less frequently. And do not assume that you are one of them...in all probability you're not.

If I have learned anything in my nine years of experience with and observations of individuals training in commercial gyms it is this: even if you possess a near god-like physique, an astounding recovery ability, and a psyche of laser-like focus, *you will* eventually become too damn strong to recover from your workouts and you will plateau, hit a sticking point, ride the broken escalator of development, or whatever you want to call it, unless you take specific actions to accommodate your growing strength…count on it.

However, stumbling in the blind ally of confusion, it is only natural that one would look to successful individuals for direction…but do not be deceived by wolves lurking in sleep's clothing. I give ode to the muscle magazines with their primrose promises of routines that affirm that they will "produce" the muscles you desire…but only if you consume such and such product first….While contrary to what most people believe on the subject of exercise, no amount of exercise will produce growth, only the body produces growth. And there is a specific order of actions that your body performs after a workout, if you do not interrupt the body with more exercise: first, it will start to recover the debt in its resources and then, only after the body has recovered first, will it begin the process of increasing muscular size…and even that is not instantaneous. When training, you must train infrequently enough that you allow both time to recover and then for additional growth, and for about 80 percent of the population, training once every five to seven days is ideal, initially…10 percent are a rare few who can tolerate more with great results…the other 10 percent are individuals that will require even less frequency… considerably less.

Theoretical knowledge

Man, by his nature, is required to be a rational being in order for him to survive. We have evolutionarily traded the natural brute strength of other beings of the hominidae biological family for an, up till now, unimaginable intellectual ability. Human beings possess the faculty of reason, to be exact, the capability of reason, not the automatic innate ability. We have the ability to choose: choose to create or destroy, choose to try to understand or just to disregard, choose to flee or to fight! Our defining human characteristic is that we are required to choose, not through instinct, but through a volitional choice.

Every individual has the irrefutable human right and ability to choose to think or not, to accept or not and to act or not. This book is neither an order to think nor to accept the information within it. It is only on the basis of grasping an argument that one should agree or not. The ability to apply the scientific objective principles on how to hypertrophy the muscular tissues of the human body is the choice that every individual has. However, as you continue on reading this book you will be further inundated with facts of the human body that will have you questioning the socially accepted lifestyle of a bodybuilder as being a socially benign gym rat.

The theory of high intensity training is as scientifically valid and as universally objective as Isaac Newton's laws of motion, Robert Hooke's cell theory and Charles Darwin's theory of evolution. The theory of high intensity training is in fact the only theory qua theory of bodybuilding exercise, as a theory is a set of abstract principles, logically connected, which purports to be either a correct description of some aspect of reality and/or a guideline for successful human action.

Since all other training ideologies are constituted of free-floating abstractions and anti-concepts—not having referents within reality and no definition, originating from irrationality—they emerge to contradict themselves as well as each other and are thus instantaneously revealed as invalid, as Aristotle revealed: reality has no contradictions.

In fact, not only are these training methodologies composed of unintelligible bile, but they are not even theories on bodybuilding exercise, as a scientific theory (bodybuilding being a branch of medical science), to quote Thomas Paine, "has for its basis a system of principles as fixed and unalterable as those by which the universe is regulated and governed. Man cannot make principles; he can only discover them." These methods do not even build-up to the quantifiable definition of a theory since they explain nothing and they are founded upon speculation and arbitrary notions, such as tradition and feeling. They do not tell you how or why high volume (not to mention explosive training and all other erroneous styles of training) stimulates muscle growth. They never explain the mechanism in high volume training… although I suppose that it is implicitly the volume that they ascribe to be the cause…but refer to my comparison between the sprinter and marathon runner earlier and you will see the insanity in such a notion.

The contention of their high volume rhetoric, that is, how and what is required for muscle to grow is that muscle is some *"je ne sais quoi."* They reassure you that, "Everyone is different and requires a different, *uniquely individual*, style of training." Only to follow-up with (contradicting themselves in the process) a "universal" routine stating that you must perform such and such exercises, such and such times for the majority of the week.

Not surprisingly, the majority of the exercise scientists, publishing provocative literature against *certainty* in the bodybuilding scientific world, will respond to the theory of high intensity training with the Platonic mind and body dichotomy assertion that, "It may be good in theory, but it doesn't work in practice." To this I quote Ayn Rand from her book *Philosophy: Who Needs It.*

"What is a theory? It is a set of abstract principles purporting to be either a correct description of reality or a set of guidelines for man's actions. Correspondence to reality is the standard of value by which one estimates a theory. If a theory is inapplicable to reality, by what standards can it be estimated as "good"? If one were to accept that notion, it would mean: a. that the activity of man's mind is unrelated to reality, b. that the purpose of thinking is neither to acquire knowledge nor to guide man's actions. (The purpose of that catch phrase is to invalidate man's conceptual faculty.)"

Is it any wonder why the world encompassing, not only bodybuilding, but all realms of intellectual and moral pursuit are cascading into an obfuscating abyss—with "experts," embracing a pragmatic philosophy, raping all fields of intellectual thought. Philosophies purporting ineffable, arbitrary speculative vomit as man's only means of finding truth and happiness (platonic), or even rejecting these concepts as being unattainable by man; that man is incapable of gaining knowledge and possessing certainty—that man is forever damned (Kantian). Understand reader that since there *is* only one reality there can only possibly be one immutably correct theory on any aspect of it; whether it is productive bodybuilding exercise, mathematics, physics, evolution.

In order to grasp such vital information man requires valid theoretical knowledge.

However, theoretical knowledge derived from the imagination, apart from reality, and attempted to be rationalized into reality (such is what the majority of scientists today are doing) is worse than worthless. Worse because it spreads misinformation instead of nothing at all...ignorance is usually safe, people who don't know what to do usually just don't do anything that could lead to an accident...but stupidity, when people are misinformed and believe that they know the answers when they do not even have the slightest clue, that gets people killed. The theoretical is derived from the metaphysical for the purpose of comprehending the concrete to a greater degree, not from the irrational ejaculation of the imagination into an idea that is so deeply coveted by the person that they relentlessly endeavor with the impossibility of fitting it into the real world—rationalization. Our ivory tower intellectuals start with the answers they want to hear and make up the questions and equations to justify them. I believe that Nikola Tesla stated the situation in the sciences perfectly when he stated... "Today's scientists have substituted mathematics for experiments, and they wander off through equation after equation, and eventually build a structure which has no relation to reality."

4

Individual Potential

"The only way most people recognize their limits is by trespassing on them."

Tom Morris

The Human body is an astonishing universe of matter that is dazzling with its innumerable chemical reactions and potential reactions that lay dormant until some unique stimulus has been introduced to ignite such tremendous biological fireworks.

Beautiful in its conception, brought about by the resilience and combination of breeding, evolution and the actions of one's ancestral parents, every individual is magnificently conceived with their endowed physical potentialities that are uniquely given to them and them alone.

Therefore, it goes to say that, no one individual can be compared equally to any other individual on any basis of strength, height or even intellect for a matter of fact, due to the influence of two immense factors, of which, only one you have control over. These factors pertain to one's history; which generally grouped are: environment, volitional actions i.e.: diet, drug use, willingness to gain knowledge, etc. The larger of these two influences, more influential in many respects, is the second unalterable characteristic of an individual's genetic endowment. The first factor I touch upon in other chapters of this book and how they influence your physical and intellectual stature. In this chapter however, I will illustrate the capabilities of the human being's primary genetic factors that influence every aspect of your physical ability.

Comparing Genetics

Every individual's physical and intellectual potential is predisposed within a limited continuum. The range of such continuum is set within the physical and intellectual parameters of characteristic potentialities of the human species. If you were to graph the entirety of humanity, or simply your city and its population's genetic endowment you would observe the result of a bell-shaped curve. On this curve, you would see that the majority of your city or the entirety of humanity is disposed in the center, with a significantly small minority of individuals being conceived into either of the two extremes of such a graph. We also observe that this bell-shaped curve resides in all aspects of genetic endowment.

This is most readily available to observe with individual ranges of height and intelligence. With height you have a significantly few individuals who are midget in stature and on the other end of that same spectrum you have incredible eight-foot giants. With regards to intelligence, you have individuals that are medical morons, lacking the basic ability to perform even basic arithmetic of one plus one, contrasted with fantastic geniuses on the other end being able to grasp and perform such spectacular intellectual feats such as performing advanced trigonometry in their heads.

The same continuum applies to muscular capability. This can be seen with the atypical high ranked bodybuilder or athlete with his naturally low body fat level, extremely well developed muscularity and a solid, large frame with chiseled features and his ability to display extraordinary physical competence and muscular prowess...as against the atypical scrawny bodybuilder that has been training, eating and practicing in the same fashion—or even better in all these aspects—and for just as long as the Herculean muscled bodybuilder, but their growth is less than modest at best and cannot muscularly keep up with the rest of the competition no matter how hard they try.

We find by means of a process of elimination through visual observation that there is a myriad of physical dissimilarities between the massive and the scrawny bodybuilder. It becomes brazenly valid to note that this later individual of lesser prowess just genetically cannot possibly compete on an equal plane of comparative physiques among the gifted bodybuilder. But why is this so?

It is because his genetic makeup is not intended for performing exceedingly well in that type of physical endeavor; in either following the set accordance of neuromuscular movements (this pertains to skills required in sports) or not being able to put forth the competitively required muscular size.

Genetics are a seemingly infinitely complex spectrum of study, with so many variables and having so many factors that contribute to one's physical potential that vary in importance from parental heredity to random mutations of chromosomes. However, in this chapter we will only concern ourselves with some of the best-known and studied factors that determine one's muscular size and strength potential.

Muscle Belly Length

The most readily available, and a reasonably accurate, way of assessing an individual's physical potential is their muscle belly length. Muscle belly length is the distance end to end of a muscle. Muscle belly length is contingent on the ratio between muscular tissue and its corresponding tendon that anchors the muscle into its point of insertion. The length of the muscle in relation to the tendon is the ultimate factor in one's muscle size/strength potential if all other genetic factors are in generous endowment. As a muscle's width will never exceed its length, which means that the longer the muscle, the greater its potential for acquiring mass.[1]

The factor of length is huge in assessing a muscle's functional potential. There is a definite aspect ratio that a muscle can never transcend; an aspect ratio of 1 to 1 would be the absolute limit, because anything over that would make the muscle incapable of functioning properly. An aspect ratio of 1 to 1 means that if a muscle was 4 inches in length, it has the ultimate potential (if generously endowed with all other muscle size factors) of a width of 4 inches. Few individuals actually appreciate the gain of an inch on the circumference of their upper arms…but only a fool would still under appreciate such a monumental achievement after grasping the facts of the matter.

If an individual started the training program outlined in this book with a triceps length of six inches and a width of two inches and, through six months of intense training, increased the width of his triceps muscle to six inches this individual would have produced a degree of growth that few would not desire.

The cross-section of his triceps muscle (if is was a quadrangle and we treat it without introducing any error for calculations sake) at the beginning of this program was 12 square inches (two by six), but after six months of intense training he increased the muscular cross-section area of his triceps to 36 square inches (six by six), tripling the cross-section mass of his triceps...but in reality, the increase is size would be much greater than this since we are not dealing with two dimensions but three. His former mass would be approximately 24 inches cubed (two by two by six)...after increasing the width of his triceps muscle three fold his actual gain is of the order of 216 squared inches (six by six by six), increasing his triceps mass by 800 percent...but such an increase in mass would result in approximately two to three inches increase in the circumference of his upper arm...and even less for an individual who already possesses large arms. So now it should be clear that an individual with an upper arm that has increased in circumference from training by one or two inches has by no means accomplished a trivial feat.

One factor about muscle growth that is also fairly unknown to most is that, once a muscle reaches a certain point in size, every increase in size actually weakens the ratio of capable force of the muscle to actual output force able to be produced. Why? It is due to a change in shape.

When something increases in size to a certain extent, it invariably has to change its shape in order to maintain a specific function: can you imagine the Burj Dubai with the shape of the CN Tower or a supergiant sauropod dinosaur like Argentinosaurus with a vertebra the same shape and size of that of a cow…certainly not. A muscle's ratio of actual strength to output strength degrades as a muscle grows in size because as a muscle changes its shape it changes its angle of pull. Only the muscle fibers that are located exactly on the centerline of the muscle are capable of pulling in exactly the right direction; while any other muscle fibers that are above, below or to the side of the exactly centerline will not be pulling in the same direction. Thus, some muscle fibers will not be as effective as others are when you are trying to contract that muscle against a form of resistance.

So what does this mean? It means that the larger your muscle becomes the smaller the increases in strength will be. So, if you are in possession of a few rather long muscle bellies, as these muscles reach close to their full potential, something as incremental as a five pound increase in your strength will represent a significant change.

But now on to the most important issue with muscle belly length: when it comes to attaining tremendous degrees in muscular size and strength, why is it that some individuals can and many others cannot? Why does a small difference in length make such a difference in size and strength potential?

While it is true that nobody knows just what the maximum aspect ratio of a muscle is—and I will not even consider the grotesque physical state of individuals pumped up with synthol oil—it is obvious that there does exist a definite limitation. And it is also obvious that if a muscle is longer than average, then it will have the maximum potential to increase its width directly proportional to its abnormal length.

To quote Arthur Jones on this issue… "The potential cross-section of the muscle does not increase in direct proportion; in fact, the resulting increase in muscular cross-section will be much greater than might be expected. If the muscle's length is twice as great as average, this means that its maximum width is also twice as great as average, but that its maximum cross-section is four times as great as average, and that its maximum 'mass' (or overall size) is eight times as great as average. Thus it follows that having muscles that are even slightly longer than average gives you the potential of greatly increased muscular size."

Stating all of the above, I am not implying that one has the capability to *increase* the length of their muscle bellies, you don't—contrary to what the bodybuilding magazines and personal trainers try to tell you. Your various muscle lengths were determined even before your conception—they're hereditary, just like all other physical characteristics.

The length of any specific muscle seems to be a random feature within any given individual's musculature, with differences usually existing from one body part to the next. It is only the extremely rare individual who has uniform muscle length over his entire body[2]—individuals such as Sergio Oliva and Flex Wheeler are not your typical human beings. However, if you do not have particularly long muscle bellies in your biceps and/or your triceps do not worry, that does not mean that every muscle is that way in your body. The general population is a varied mix of everything between long and short lengths over the genetic bell shaped curve. Yet, even with average or short muscle bellies, it does not invariably mean that you will not be able to develop a very impressive degree of muscular mass...other factors, less obvious to the eye, have the potential of producing great size.

Muscle Structure

An enormous factor in one's muscular size potential is the structure of which a particular muscle takes. For example, the biceps of the upper arm or the vastus medialis of the quadriceps are generally structured like a football with the vast majority of their mass residing in the center, with a tendon attached to both ends. Owing to their three-dimensional structure, these types of muscles possess great size potential. These muscle fiber structures are set in a group called fusiform muscle fibers.

The contrasting group of structures on the other end of the spectrum are found when we look at the muscles of the hands and the feet. These muscles are only a few fibers thick, with a feather like structure and are setup in a mechanically leverage advantageous position—able to produce maximal direct contractile ability and generate enormous amounts of contractile force. Because of their two dimensional shape this group of structures have a significantly low hypertrophy potential, but still possess enormous strength potential relative to their size. These are classed into a group of muscle fiber structures known as pennate muscle fibers.

There exists an entire spectrum of muscle fiber

arrangements between these two extremes, and in a given muscle group different individuals might have a more fusiform, or a more pennate fiber arrangement.[3] As we see with muscle belly length, everyone is usually a mixture of some sorts, with rare genetic anomalies presenting themselves to the world in very low frequencies.

Cross-Section Fiber Density

Let us say that you possess an extraordinary genetic endowment in the length of all your muscle bellies and have an extremely high percentage of muscles that are fusiform in structure. Should we assume that you are in possession of a physique that will grow far beyond man's imagination of muscularity and strength? Well sorry to say this, but you are not out of the woods yet my friend. To analogize this in a more industrial approach, say that you are building a skyscraper with the base set: having the rebar set, the footings dug, the concrete poured, spread and dried, etc.—this will represent muscle belly length, as you are restricted in the height of the tower by the amount of land available to you.

You also have the architect's blueprints of the marvel to be—this will represent muscle structure. Finally, we will have a certain extent of materials to be used for the skeletal structure, the floors, walls, and so-on—representing fiber muscle density. Now, if you are building a skyscraper and run out of available material, you are not able to go any farther than that point…are you. You cannot reach the full potential that was laid out for you by your muscle belly length.

Fiber density is the number of muscle fibers in any

given cross-sectional area of a muscle. Fiber density, like muscle length, determines the mass potential of a muscle. The more muscle fibers per given volume of a muscle, the thicker that muscle's potential to develop.[4]

Yet, muscle fiber density may not be set in stone for every individual from birth. There is great debate over the possibility of the phenomenon known as *Hyperplasia*. A concept that means instead of the growth and thickening of a muscle fiber (Hypertrophy) they split and divide or fuse myogenic stem cells (satellite cells) creating new muscle fibers, producing a more fiber dense cross-section area.

There have been some documented cases in which physiologists have induced the first form of hyperplasia in lower order animals. But! And I want to strongly emphasize this, there has been *no* evidence whatsoever that it can occur in primates.

There is, although, good evidence that new muscle fibers can be generated from myogenic stem cells that exist within a muscle. With a high intensity stimulus these cells can possibly be activated and differentiate into new muscle cells which increase fiber density and can undergo hypertrophy and contribute to increased mass.[5] So an individual with a large number of satellite cells and average muscle fiber density might have larger size and strength potential if they are able to stimulate the fusion of myogenic stem cells through high intensity training.

Muscle Fiber Type

The length of the muscle belly, its fiber density, metabolism, skeletal structure and countless more that

I will not get into, due to their less import, determine potential for great athletic ability and muscular size. An athlete needs to be able to perform under specific circumstances that their sport demands. If you are a successful competitive marathon runner, required by your sport to run for very long periods with little or no rest, your body has wondrously adapted to that type of activity. Or say you are an accomplished sprinter or swimmer, required to reach a short distance very quickly, your body has adapted to these circumstances. But how is it possible that some individuals will perform exceedingly well in one realm of activity, but not in the other…why can't they have both ultra endurance and super strength?

It is primarily due to these individuals' muscle fiber type dominance. All of your muscles have within them several different types of fibers; any given muscle has within it a mixed conglomeration of muscle fiber types that can differ tremendously from individual to individual and even from muscle to muscle within the same individual. Although there are many types of muscle fiber, they can be narrowed down into four separate categories:

Type I or SO	Slow, Oxidative
Type IIa or FO	Fast, Oxidative; FR (Fast, Fatigue Resistant
Type IIab or FOG	Fast, Oxidative-Glycolytic; FI (Fast, Intermediate Fatigueability
Type IIb or FG	Fast, Glycolytic; FF (Fast, Fatigueable)

We possess within all of us these muscle fibers in different quantities, unique for each muscle throughout our bodies. Most sports trainers and some fitness trainers believe that there are only two dominate categories of muscle fiber: red, branded as being slow twitch, and white, known as fast twitch. From that, they conclude that since one is "slow" and the other is "fast" you need to train each fiber type uniquely by performing fast cadence movements, performed for very few repetitions or slow cadenced movements, performed in great numbers of repetitions for long durations, in order to train the two specifically.

This dated pseudo-scientific notion that asserts that you have to train the fast twitch muscle fibers by performing a fast, explosive movement is not only incorrect but also pure stupidity…it is utterly insane. On the other hand, the performance of light and long duration exercises, performed for countless sets is, at best, only a waste of time and, at worst, leaves you so overtrained that your muscular tissue starts to decompensate; the muscle lacks a sufficient stimulus for hypertrophying, yet is still being drained of resources. In reality, being fast or slow twitch has little to do with their speed, but with their fatigueability. The greater the initial power a muscle fiber can exert, the quicker the fiber fatigues.

For simplicity's sake, we will divide the muscle fibers into three categories: slow twitch (greater endurance, but lowest hypertrophy/strength potential), intermediate twitch (moderate endurance, moderate hypertrophy/strength potential) and fast twitch (low endurance, but high hypertrophy/strength potential). The actual means to activate a muscle fiber type is via motor unit recruitment.

A motor unit is a group of homogenous muscle fibers bundled together randomly throughout a given muscle. A motor unit has a muscle neuron that receives signals from the brain via the central nervous system. When a nerve impulse is received by a motor neuron it will activate that motor unit to contract in an *all or nothing* fashion. This is true for all motor units—once activated they will contract with 100 percent intensity or not at all.

So, in view of the fact that a muscle fiber will contract in an "all or nothing" fashion, why do we not remove flesh when scratching our forearm or break the spine of an infant when we are burping them? It is because *a muscle will only contract with the least amount of motor units necessary to perform any given task*. At the start, a muscle will activate only the lower order—slow twitch—motor units. But once they fatigue and become unable to perform the given task your muscles will recruit the next order of motor units that fatigue faster, but are stronger than the previous ones—the intermediate. Then, if only exposed to a significant enough load and intensity, you will fatigue the intermediate fibers and require the recruitment of the highest order, the strongest motor units—fast twitch. And after fatiguing the fast twitch motor units, you will reach momentary muscular failure.

This sequential recruitment of muscle fibers can occur at an incredible rate; being as fast a one to six seconds—however, if you are exposing a muscle to a load that requires it to exert itself maximally right off the hop, you will recruit all of the muscle fibers at once, doing so, you will exhaust the fast twitch fibers immediately, not allowing the lower order intermediate and slow twitch fiber to fatigue, thus you will not develop that muscle maximally by stimulating all of the fibers possible.

This being understood, the muscle's muscle fiber or motor unit composition now comes in to questioning. How do I tell if I have a predominance slow or fast twitch motor units? There is an answer to this question, but it is very painful. A muscle biopsy is an option…but I would not recommend it. The procedure of a muscle biopsy requires having a long, thick needle inserted into the muscle belly (usually the vastus head of the quadriceps), cutting a column of living muscular tissue and then removing it from the muscle for analysis—all-around, not a very pleasant procedure. However, later on I will go into further detail about the implications of muscle fiber type in your training program and a fairly accurate method of assessing your fiber type predominance.

Neuromuscular Efficiency

Though it may be incredible to consider, it is virtually impossible to involve the entire mass of any skeletal muscle in a normal contraction. This simply means that, an average individual never uses more than a rather small percentage of any muscle at any point in time. Even in most maximal life and death struggles (e.g. a mother lifting a turned over car a few inches to save their child), only part of any muscle is being used…while the remainder of the muscle, the largest section, is inactive.

But if this is true, one might ask, what purpose does the extra unusable bulk of muscle serve? The extra muscular mass in fact serves a very important purpose… it provides muscular endurance. Furthermore, it actually is usable, but not in concert with the rest of the muscle in a normal contraction.

Understand that if all of the fibers in any given muscle were fired simultaneously, the resulting force would be so tremendous that the muscle would almost certainly be torn free from the bones that it is attached or the bones themselves might shatter instead, not snap in half, but quite literally longitudinally compact like a pop can. Some individuals who survive accidental electrocution suffer broken bones and torn muscles or connective tissues as a direct result of the violent muscular contractions that are produced by a powerful electrical stimulation.

In any given moment, a fresh, rested muscle is capable of contracting 100 percent of its fibers simultaneously... however, the nervous system is not. A muscular contraction is triggered by an electrical impulse from the nervous system, yet there are not enough nerves available to stimulate all of the fibers at the same time. Because of this, the average individual is only capable of contracting 30 percent of any given muscle all at once.

Despite this fact, it does not follow that all individuals are thus the same, a few uncommon individuals are capable of contract as much as 40 percent of the same muscle, and a few exceedingly rare individuals can contract up to 50 percent of the muscle.

This means, in practical terms, that some men are far stronger than other men are, with all other genetic factors being equal. But it also means that these stronger-than-average individuals, with higher than average neuromuscular efficiency, have less than an average amount of muscular endurance—not cardiovascular endurance, which has absolutely nothing to do with the matter.

The ability to contract a high percentage of fibers increases a muscle's power potential, thus enabling more powerful muscular contractions, thus facilitating greater strength and speed. In terms of endurance, this is a disadvantage, but it is a great advantage for stimulating muscle growth or single attempt efforts.

If you desire to witness such extremes in neuromuscular efficiency, take a look at Olympic sprinters. These individuals have a neuromuscular efficiency close to 50 or 60 percent. At this level of capability, it is no wonder why so many tear hamstrings and quadriceps, when they are generating so much force.

Skeletal Structure

The ability to possess large quantities of muscle mass is most predominantly determined by one's skeletal structure. The size and formation of an individual's bones dictates how much muscle can be carried or supported by those bones, in addition to determining muscle shape and density, two factors that impart an aesthetic quality to a physique.[6] Evolutionarily it would be a disadvantage for individuals with larger skeletal frames to possess a diminutive magnitude of muscular mass, being at a leverage disadvantage it is usually balanced with greater strength, though that is not always the case.

Strength potential is hugely determined by bone length and its formation. Compare two very well developed individuals: one being 6 feet 6 inches tall and the other being 5 feet 6 inches. We will assert that they can both curl 200 pounds for one maximum repetition in a standing barbell curl. You could speculate and draw the conclusion that these two individuals are equal in strength in that particular lift. However, that is where you would be wrong. The taller individual will—ignoring genetic osteological malformations present in a few rare individuals—have ulna and radius bones of their forearms that are much longer than those of the shorter individual.

Now for that reason, the taller individual must generate greater power in order to move the same load as the shorter individual. Because of this, the taller individual's biceps are both exposed to this stress over a longer range, thus needing to have stronger biceps in order to finish the full range of the exercise, and he is lifting a heavier load than the shorter individual is because of his leverage disadvantage—there is greater torque. The latter is easily demonstrated with trying to lift a person on an opposing end of a teeter-totter by pushing down close to the middle. The closer you go towards the center, the harder it becomes as you are required to produce a greater force to equal the foot-pounds of force opposing since you are shortening your moment arm or lever.

When we are assessing an individual's predisposition towards building a championship physique, it is essential to consider bodily proportions, which are determined by the length, thickness, and ratio of an individual's bones.[7] When you look at most professional bodybuilders, hockey players or sprinters you will notice that their wrists are usually thicker than average and their shoulders are usually wider. They have the skeletal structure needed in order to allow them their exceptional musculature.

Metabolism

A critical factor in one's ability to develop muscle tissue is their metabolism. We have all witnessed individuals in the gym with a nearly perfect physique, who perform demanding workouts, eating anything and everything under the sun, and develop to degrees that are just too damn impressive for words. We have all also seen the contrast of this chiseled Greek Gods with the individuals in the gym who look as if they were afflicted with a muscle wasting disease—individuals that seem to be able to eat like a starved elephant, but can barely maintain their body weight as it is.

Metabolically, some individuals are geared towards building large muscles more than others are. One's metabolism is alterable to a finite degree with dietary modification—that can dramatically affect your hormone profile and promote your production of anabolic hormones—and intense physical activity—that alters numerous hormones and redirects nutrients among tissues of the body. Though individuals do possess the ability to control their internal environment to a desirable state, there still exists the genetically predetermined degree of improvability that is finite, that is, some individuals will produce tremendous muscular size with proper dieting and training and others may have the predisposition of someone like Woody Allen.

And odds are that you are neither one of either of these two individuals—neither blessed with almost superhuman potential nor accursed with a meager potential of growth. But even so, *everyone* will progress to a tremendous degree, far more than with any other method, with the implementation of the only rational and sane method of exercise there is, which just so happens to be high intensity training.

Genetic Health

Genetics play the definitive role in a muscle's size and strength potential, but this is just scratching the surface of the role that genetics plays in our lives. Since the whole of my work is focused on "bodybuilding"—I place the word bodybuilding in quotations in an attempt to emphasize what my research and practices are directed towards: the understanding and building of the body (and the brain is apart of the body and the mind is a product of the brain)—I have made it my key concern in life to understand how one is able to improve their body, including their mind, in the most efficacious manner possible. Bodybuilding, in a historical context, is the improvement of oneself, including their intellect and their longevity of their capability to participate in the activities that they hold so dear to them—e.g. playing with their children or even great grandchildren, spending time with their friends, playing with their pets, having a romantic relationship and so on. This, in my opinion, is the greatest gift that one could ever give their self. This is the most selfish thing one can do: the pursuing of happiness.

Genetics predisposes people to a health potential that is, generally, unchangeable; with diseases and immunity to disease engraved into your DNA at conception. The first thing I would like to state is that exercise of any kind will not improve health beyond your genetics, contrary to what everyone thinks. In general, most people who are healthy and frequently exercise are not healthy because they exercise. Usually, they exercise because they are healthy.[8] Exercise is actually killing many people all over the world!

This has to do with recovery ability, which I will get into next. However, understand that before the industrial revolution the average life expectancy was around 47 years. One could say that they were exposed to disease and did not have very effective, or any, medicine at the time. This may be true, but why did all these people become so susceptible to these sicknesses in the first place? Their recovery ability was the predominant deciding factor.

Every physical exertion with moderate to large amounts of biochemical resources consumed during performing their daily-activities—mining, forced labor, forestry, farming, construction, digging, etc.—consumed some percentage out of their body's *limited* reserve and, when it was not filled back up, they became more and more depleted. Depleted to a degree that resulted in either immunological vulnerability—leading to a disease like the plague or syphilis killing nearly half the population of Europe—or death by organ failure.

After the industrial revolution, the introduction of mechanical instruments started taking over the more demanding tasks, division of labor allowed individuals to specialize in the newly developed fields, instead of having to generalize in everything that was essential for a pre-industrial life—which amounted to about 18 hour days of labor, 7 days a week. The workdays got shorter and individuals were able to afford luxuries that allowed them to relax and recover. The result of this was that the average life expectancy skyrocketed and the infant/child mortality rate plummeted dramatically.

(...So the next time you want to thank someone for your longer life expectancy and your standard of living that does not require you to work 18 hours a day on the farm, and that empowers you with the opportunity to choose to live your life in nearly any fashion and in almost any endeavor you desire, don't thank your doctor, your health food store or an environmentalist—thank an industrialist, a businessman, a capitalist.)

Recovery ability is genetically predisposed and varies among individuals enormously. Some very rare individuals will simple die from their lack of ability to cope with the stresses of intense physical exertion and other, equally rare, individuals can work for 16-hour days, 6 or 7 days a week and be in amazing health, living into their hundreds.

Very few people grasp that exercise is a *negative*. It causes a loss of vital recourses that require time to replenish (the necessity of which will be discussed in the next chapter). Yet still experts cry out that daily exercise is essential for health, that people are still not doing enough exercise; even though every study that has ever tried to show that exercise improves health has only done so on a leap of faith. Every study has clearly established the association between exercise and health, but then made the leap that this association is based on causation without further understanding their relationship.

But, if you take each one of these studies and skip over the parts that everyone reads (the abstract and the conclusion), and read the part that nobody reads (the methods section), you will find something that every single one of these studies contains—selection bias.[9] The only thing one can do to fight off their genetic reaper to the extent that possible for them is to have a caloric intake that is not at a surplus that is not required for muscle tissue development and making sure they obtain a balance diet with the four basic food groups and a little of the sweets they love, in appropriate amounts for psychological gratification. However, one more factor can better your health to its maximum…increase your muscle mass. Simply put, greater muscle mass sustained over one's life allows them greater functional capability. (For more information on how vital muscle is for your life, consult some of Dr. Doug McGuff's articles or his new book, co-authored with John Little, *Body by Science.*)

The development of a muscle improves its function. A muscle's main function is to produce force, but the purpose of this function is to pull the area where the muscle inserts into towards the muscle's origin of attachment through that particular muscle's intended potential range of motion.

Therefore, this means that your flexibility is genetically predisposed too. Flexibility is a genetically predetermined variable that can only reach its full potential from exercise, as you are improving its function. But in order to elicit this increased functional ability the exercises must become stronger through full-range intense exercise. The stretching that people complain that they are lacking in a high intensity training program is actually built into the exercise. A definition of stretching that most of the stretching orthodoxy throng would agree upon is that stretching is the application of force on a muscle in its extreme range of motion. Well, during a proper set of high intensity exercise you are moving through a full-range of motion—this includes the fully extended position—, moving a significant load, or force, from the fully contracted position to the fully extended position. Obtaining a significant and far safer stretch in the fully extended position, allowing you to at least keep or increase your flexibility while becoming stronger. A strength that actually allows you to reach such ranges of motion, though many still attribute the *false* premise of stretching improving flexibility instead of the *fact* that only when a muscle is strong enough can it reach such ranges of motion. Proper strength training will increase your flexibility to its optimal potential without relying on damaging the joints and connective tissues....Damage that is required to permit those extreme ranges of motion performed in yoga and other stretching activities.

Recovery Ability

The genetic factor that plays the definitive role in the rate of your muscle growth and your entire physiologic development is your recovery ability. The subject of recovery ability is misunderstood greatly by the majority of humanity and, as a result, has created a massive health crisis in our Western world. Arthur Jones once said that if you were to rate the physical fitness of all the people in America from one to ten it would probably be a negative four...if everybody stopped performing what they thought was exercise, what they believed was "beneficial," that rating would rise to zero. And if you have honestly taken a look at the state of America today, the school gym classes, the fitness centers, the individuals running on the road, wheezing as if they are trying to breathe through a toothpick, you would not be one to hastily disagree with that statement.

One must grasp that it is one's recovery ability that is the ultimate factor in their ability to live or die from the imposition of a certain totality of stress imposed upon them, whether it is imposed physiologically or psychologically.

When dealing with the issue of recovery ability we are inadvertently dealing with the subject of energy. And energy is the most precious thing in the universe. Without energy the planets would not rotate, the sun would cool and become dead and motionless; there would be no light, no heat and no life. Our bodies, just as the sun, the earth and the universe, possess a finite supply of energy—only having a limited amount of resources to draw upon. Life requires energy to merely sustain itself and more so to grow—bodybuilders need not be reminded that they require energy to maintain their workouts and require more energy to build muscle.

This energy comes from the sun's spectrum of radiations, from the food we eat and the air we breathe. However, just because you are exposed to these forms of energy does not mean that your body will utilize them instantaneously. In order to use these forms of energy requires time for your body to process them. And since we are trying to create new living tissue, it is not surprising that this process requires generous amounts of time and a notable sum of resources. Yet many bodybuilders ignore this former fact and continue exercising without allowing time for their body's recuperative subsystems to merely compensate for the demands of their workouts, let alone time for muscle growth to manifest.

(A training program that does not take the trainee's recovery ability into consideration will not only prevent or retrogress their muscle growth, but may actually be harming them. As I said previously, exercise is literally killing people, and this is why.)

How much an activity depletes one's energy reserves is contingent upon the intensity needed to conduct such an activity and/or the volume or quantity of the activity performed. And since we are pursuing muscular growth we are required to perform exercises of an extremely intense nature, because of which, we create an enormous debt of our biochemical reserves. I quote Mike Mentzer from John Little and Joanne Sharkey's *The Wisdom of Mike Mentzer.*

"If you were to draw a horizontal line from left to right across a page of paper with that line representing zero effort and then off of that line graph your average daily effort output the graph representing that kind of effort output would barely leave the flat line; it would be a little squiggly sine wave. Then all of a sudden you do into the gym and you perform a heavy set of partial bench presses or a set of heavy Nautilus laterals, whatever, all of a sudden that little squiggly line starts to take off in a straight vertical line off the paper, out the door, down the street, and around the block! Now within that space is how much more biochemical resources are used up."

You must understand that the human body possesses only 100 units of adaptation energy—the quantity of yours is dependent upon your genetics and minimally by your training. If you are performing any demanding tasks, in either intensity or duration, you use a certain quantity of those 100 units. If are performing aerobics for a fair period of time, multiple times a week, not allowing time for a replenishment of the certain quantity of adaptive energy utilized, you see that it may not be as "healthy" as once thought. Moreover, if this is done in concert with intense weight lifting exercise you run the risk of overtraining even more so.

Realize that the human body does not possess 100 units of adaptation energy for aerobics, sports or social activities and 100 units for weight training, but merely 100 units *total*. Any slight decrease from one activity where time is not instituted for replenishment influences the whole, upon which your muscle growth is abruptly obstructed of maximal gains.

This by absolutely no means implies that an individual is to be constrained from all physical exertion outside the gym for muscle gains. However, in order to optimize muscle growth the individual should accommodate their body's recovery ability with sufficient replenishment of its stores: in essence, do not perform any activity that has a value to be gained in a haphazard manner. (For example, if you are competing in hockey or football tournaments keep in mind that these activities physically drain you immensely.)

How long does it take a person to completely recover from a workout and then overcompensate with a gain in muscle size and strength? Well this is not a simple question to answer. Using high intense exercise as the form of intense stress, I will try to explain the severity of debt that intense weight training can produce.

"My data, collected on the subject at my training

facility, showed a slight response at 48-72 hours, adequate at about 4 days and very good for most at 7 days. In my opinion, something between 5-7 days is a good starting point. (In retrospect, I can now say anything more frequent than working out more than once a week will constitute overtraining for about 95 percent of the population).[10]"

Doug McGuff, MD—writer of the above quote—, at his training facility *Ultimate Exercise*, took his clients to *only* positive momentary muscular failure. The significance of being only positive failure is that the human muscular system possesses three types of strength. The first is the positive or lifting the weight, of which is the weakest, due to the fact that you are not only contracting against the resisting force of the weight you are lifting, but in addition to the opposing internal friction of the muscles and joints being used in that movement (anything that has mass and motion has friction). The second type of strength is the static or the holding of the weight, which is stronger than the positive, as you are purely contracting against only the load and not against internal friction as well. The last and the strongest muscular strength is the negative or lowering of the weight. This strength is the strongest because, in an addition to the muscles contracting against the load, you also have internal friction working *with you*, making it easier to lower it than it was to lift—I will further discuss the matter and importance of muscular friction in a later chapter. When you bring one type of strength to failure, you create a certain drain upon your energy reserves proportionate to the inroad in your maximal strength. The stronger the type of strength, the greater the deficit when it is brought to failure.

It was demonstrated in a study that was published in the May 1993 edition of the Journal of Physiology that showed the significance of draining the strongest level of strength. The experimenters, John N. Howell, Gary Chleboun, and Robert Conaster (from the Somatic Dysfunction Research Laboratory of the Collage of Osteopathic Medicine and the Department of Biological Sciences, at Ohio University, Athens) reported that, a group of men and women aged 22 to 32 took part in an exercise experiment in which they trained their biceps in a negative-only fashion to a point of muscular failure. In the experiment, the subjects sat on a preacher curl bench and preformed three negative-only sets of preacher curls in which the resistance was raised for them, and they had to concentrate on lowering the resistance in a span of five to nine seconds. (Typically, each set consisted of five to fifteen such repetitions.)

It was undeniable the day after their three-set workout that the subjects were in no condition to train again, exhibiting what the experimenters termed "a dramatic 35 percent loss of strength." Moreover, ten days after the workout, the subjects' recovery ability was only 5 percent better, as the experimenters noted, "Even on the tenth post-exercise day the muscles had recovered only to about 70 percent of their control strength." If this rate is the "norm," then we are looking at 5 percent every ten days, and the full recovery process may take anywhere from sixty to seventy days (or longer)—after only a three-set workout for the biceps!

This shows how dramatic high intensity training

can be and why you must accommodate your recovery ability's needs! These are some considerations to keep in mind when training, understanding that your genetically predisposed recovery ability dictates how long it takes to recuperate, and ultimately what mode of exercise is required in order to increase muscular size and strength in the most efficient manner possible.

Précis

From all of the muscular size and strength regulating genetic factors that I have discussed, it is quite straightforward to conclude that the individual with the lesser ability of muscle growth is just not genetically intended for the particular physical avenue of professional bodybuilding and most competitive sports. And while it is not seen as politically correct to state that some individuals have the inherited potential to reach a plane of physical and intellectual excellence that ninety-nine percent of humanity have absolutely no capability to ever reach, them's the facts—*athletes are not made they are born*. This is not to say that this individual of lesser genetic potential cannot enjoy such activities or even be able to become quite competitive in the future with further physical and tactical development. However, this person will not be able to compete on a professional level with the genetically gifted who seize dominance in their respective fields. Your potential is written into your genes before you were even born, if you hope to do something about it you better have God as your tailor, because only by selecting parents that have a greater disposition for very large muscular size would you be able to even hope to stand with the likes of Markus Reinhardt or John Heart…but I don't see that happening anytime soon.

Does this mean that such an individual of lower than average physical potential is condemned to a sickly below average [in]ability in all physical endeavors? No….The odds of such an individual with that degree of a genetic ill disposition are far too remote to contemplate, though not impossible. The majority of human beings born—save for rare genetic abnormalities—are endowed genetically with a potential, if adequate for their own self-sustainment, which was brought forth by the requisite physiologic characteristics needed by their predecessors….Gifted in stature, everyone possesses the physical characteristics that allowed for the survival of their ancestors and *function dictates design.* or as someone once said, "There is only one way to build a wolf; and if it performs like a wolf then it will look like a wolf."

The fact of the matter is that evolution has established a hierarchy of evolutionary stratagems to eliminate the weak and amplifying the strong. The only means of your existence today is that evolution has endowed you with specific abilities or traits required to survive in situations that your forebears encountered and were required to overcome.

For an example, when we look at individuals of the Negroid race we see a physical trait that the majority possess that was resented (lacking of any intelligent grounds) by football coaches, identified as Negro calf. This is a physical characteristic in which the gastrocnomius and soleus muscles of the lower leg are very short and the tendon in which it is attached (the Achilles tendon) is very long. But why is this significant you ask?

Through the study of anthropology, when we examine the environment of the ancestral Negroid race, we observe that they derived in an extreme environment. In order to survive this race of man had to develop physical characteristics that would assist in evading predators and live through the dangers of their world. They had to pass on life promoting genetic characteristics in strong emphases in order for the next generation to survive.

In effect, they became faster, were able to endure long distance on foot and were able to develop a greater potential to jump with the development of larger than average buttocks muscles—the largest and most powerful muscles in the human body that contribute as much as 80 percent of our strength in running, jumping and exercises such as the squat and deadlift—allowing them to produce significantly greater force to move. What's more, a much smaller lower leg removes excess weight that only adds unwanted inertia from beneath their thighs, which improves their efficiency and lessens energy consumption. This is one reason why black athletes usually have greater success in athletic endeavors pertaining to speed, jumping height and distance.

*   *   *

Every individual possesses different degrees of functional ability—potential strength, speed, intelligence, height, and so on. In a quick synopsis, one's muscle growth potential is ultimately factored by their genetics. Now after reading this don't start panicking and pull your hair out wondering if you possess the genetic capability to develop the idiosyncratic physique of the level that a Mr. Universe possesses—very few of us do. If you are predisposed to a less than satisfactory endowment do not become disheartened, even with a less than stunning muscular potential, developing your muscles to their pinnacle of mass and strength will present your physique in a much more attractive light than otherwise. But, as Mike Mentzer espoused, potential is only something that can be accurately assessed in retrospect. In other words, you will never know until you get there, so give it your all and don't let a genetic disposition hold you back from reaching your full potential as a human being.

5

Overtraining

The notion of there being something that is infinite in any terms of measurement (i.e. length, weight, life, etc.) within the universe is merely a hysterical wish to evade death and circumvent reality, for there is no such thing as something being infinite. Some would condemn this bold statement as atheistic or just plain ignorance, as there are mentions of perpetual sanctuaries for the departed in nearly all religions and the term infinite is used in mathematics.

Firstly, to those of the religious occult, to be something that is immeasurable is to concede to the fact that that something that is not capable of being measured does not reside within the universe, as even the universe itself is capable of being measured—the universe being everything that exists. You cannot fix an infinite within the confines of a substantiated limit, as this is a contradiction.

Such a thing cannot exist, as an existent has the fundamental value of a certain quantity of units (i.e. minerals, mass, length, photons, lifespan, etc.) that allows it its identity. A quantity that is limitless (even space) cannot exist within the universe, as even the universe itself does not extend ad infinitum. Additionally, if people believed that such a thing were to exist beyond the length of the universe they face a contradiction: the universe encompasses everything that exists, if something is not within the universe than it does not exist (i.e. energy, matter, space and time).

On the other hand, concerning the correct use of the term infinite by mathematicians, the use of infinite in mathematics is merely used as a mathematical term to state the symbolic value of a symbol replacing a number (e.g. 2a = a + a). Infinite is only relative under the context of the symbol 'a' having the capacity to be any number, but only within a man's *intellectual* capacity to express a numerical quantity into a unit, whether their conceptual range only has the capacity to reach five units or the capacity of googolplex units. The term infinite is only valid if used as a *potentiality*, never in an actuality. To quote Leonard Peikoff from his lecture on *The philosophy of Objectivism* on this issue, "Notice that, actually, however many numbers you count, wherever you stop, you only reached that point, you only got so far . . . . That's Aristotle's point that the actual is always finite. Infinity exists only in the form of the ability of certain series to be extended indefinitely; but however much they are extended, in actual fact, wherever you stop it is finite."

Consider the fact that mathematics, physics and all scientific realms of the study of objective reality denounce the term "infinite" as being valid in the context of pertaining to anything within reality, for the simple fact that nothing within the universe is infinite. Now why do I see fit to begin a chapter on overtraining with such a seemingly arbitrary statement? This opening however is not a random explanation of objective truth; it is in actuality a conclusion, of which, the term overtraining is denounced by most as being nonexistent.

It must be understood that overtraining should be the single most concern for any individual wishing to gain muscle mass and strength. Overtraining is the single most cause for lack of progress in all athletic and bodybuilding endeavors today and, disturbingly, it is scarcely being taken seriously!

The term overtraining, by the great majority of bodybuilders (professional figures not withstanding), is viewed as something that is not applicable to everyone, only to those who are not motivated to keep going or as just being a very rare abnormality not to be taken seriously. Some will even shun the notion as something that happens only when you are in a state of malnourishment—not consuming the copious quantities of nutrients and calories as the professionals consume… supplemented with some fuzzy perception that modern supplemental science has created a panacea to facilitate the submission of such an irritating muscle building obstruction by bending the laws of causality.

Well, as I elucidated in the previous chapter, explaining the vital significance of recovery ability, every individual—with absolutely no exception—is genetically endowed with a *limited* extent of recovery capability. And as such, they are capable, in every case, of exhausting it and in doing so will result in the lurid state of being overtrained…or worse.

It is man's physiologic nature that demands the imposition of a high intensity training stress as the first necessary cause, but! that it is not sufficient cause to produce the desired results. One of man's specific physiologic characteristics dictates that the training stress must be cautiously regulated in terms of volume and frequency in order for the body to compensation for the exhaustive effects of the workout and then to make the requisite adaptations that increase muscular size and strength. If not taken into consideration, overtraining rears its retarding effect and muscle growth is dissolved in untold hours of useless, counterproductive exercise.

Still, a large number of bodybuilders and athletes stick to their guns and will declare that as long as one consumes a surplus of calories and nutrients they will be able to continue their high volume training and their ceaseless sessions of cardio. Believing that they will still gain muscle non-the-less or at least retain their current mass—desiring in this case not to be "too big." Well I am elated to be the bearer of bad news, as these individuals are remarkably mistaken, foolish, misguided, confused… they are anything but correct.

Overtraining is not a just some minor formality of overzealous exercising. Overtraining is *exactly that which prevents you from obtaining progressive results from your efforts*. Overtraining is something decidedly negative by its nature. The prefix "over" means exactly that, "over" what was the intended purpose or need…in excess, beyond need, too much etc.—in the very same manner as acknowledging that water is essential, so you decide to take a little swim in a lake and suck in as much water as possible as you dive down. Anything and everything in excess is destructive…no exceptions.

Drawing from my own personal experience of high volume training, I came upon the remarkable effects of such a philosophy, the ever reoccurring "more is better."

Being an individual on the far right of the genetic bell shaped curve (the gifted), I knew that I was able to endure and progress from extreme quantities of exercise, as I was gaining muscle on training routines lasting an hour or two, 3 to 4 times a week. Consequently, I became interested in finding just how far I could push my physical (not to mention psychological, as I soon found out) limits. At the start of this experiment, I took a body composition test in a Bodpod composition chamber, girth measurements and recorded my mood as well as my weight at the time. From then on it was up hill with volume.

I started training four to five times a week, training for 3 to 41/2 hours at a time, performing 20 to 70 sets per body part a workout—approximately 40 to 140 sets for that body part a week. In addition to all of this, I would perform one to two thousand sit-ups a day!, continuously without respite and then four hundred and fifty lying leg-raises.

In due course, I became haunted by a psychological dependency to exercise (comically it was only towards lift weights, as I have always loathed aerobics), as I would find myself making excuses to train longer: I became addicted to the stimulus, as John Little was sure to point out. If I trained faster than the workout before I would add more exercises and sets in order to leave at a familiarized time.

My progress stopped altogether half way through and I became increasingly tired and depressed, at a couple of instances I was literally crippled with indescribable abdominal pain that had me in to see the doctor as I was unable to stand with my upper-body higher than being parallel to the floor. This was accompanied with large losses in weight, even at a tremendous caloric surplus—as high as 4500 to 5000 plus calories a day, without any of the orthodox aerobic activities!

In a feeble effort to rectify of my rampant mood swings and falling weight I began decreasing the volume and frequency of my workouts, radically, and started training in the old Nautilus and Dorian Yates fashion of three to four times a week for half an hour to 45 minutes. Though I could not even continue on this, so I continued to reduce to Mike Mentzer's split routine as described in his last book, *High Intensity Training the Mike Mentzer Way*. Still, my progress was minimal and by the time a year had passed I felt slightly better than the few months prior, but I was still feeling as though I was perpetually tired and I was still having mild mood swings. Taking a body composition test I became incredulous…my body weight was exactly the same as it was one year prior, but my body composition had changed, drastically. In the course of one year, I lost eleven pounds of muscle tissue and gained the exact lost in body fat! And this too was from the ages of seventeen to eighteen, the time where a male is supposed to be at their pinnacle of vitality and recovery ability. From the cessation of the high volume training it took me approximately eight months to actually begin progressing again at a normal rate!

* * *

The average human being's recovery ability should not be thought as being infinite or inexhaustible, but as finite and precious. The individuals that promote high volume training in the muscle magazines, who are actually reaping muscle gains, are the genetically gifted bodybuilders, who, already genetically predisposed with abnormal recovery ability, are also using nightmarish quantities of steroids, growth hormone and countless other ever-emerging substances that even the creators do not understand. The non-steroid using bodybuilder on the other hand, the ones that these voluminous routines are being pushed on, possess natural recuperative abilities that are painstakingly slow for most, but even more so the process of additional muscular growth, for which can be negligible in some cases and nonexistent with most individuals that perform the routines prescribed by the professionals.

The term overtraining, to reiterate, is something decidedly negative; it is that which prevents you from gaining. When you consume something over what is required you are not left with the action or substance merely cancelling out itself and becoming inert, there is a negative consequence that varies in degree from the extent of your over performance or use. If you overdose on a drug, there will be a negative consequence that can harm you and even kill you. Some of the unconsidered additional dangers of overtraining were...ironically... discovered by the arch-advocate of high-volume training, Dr. Kenneth Cooper, MD. The man whom coined the phrase of "Aerobics".

In the mid 90's Dr. Cooper was astonished when he found that many of his longtime clients were developing cancer and heart disease. There were so many in fact that he became alarmed. As a result, he and several of his colleges began researching to find if there was a correlated cause for their conditions. He studied the life styles and activities of these individuals and found that they all ate balanced diets, consumed little fat, did not drink or smoke, and ran 4 to 5 times a week...even weight trained several times a week. Dr. Cooper discovered that these individuals' bodies were succumbing to over-training and because of which, began developing cancer and heart disease, among other things. The deaths of Boston Celtics star Reggie Lewis and the long-time friend of Dr. Cooper, marathon runner Jim Fixx were attributed to overtraining.

Dr Cooper ascribed the cause of the coronary disease that befell his friend Jim Fixx to the extreme production of free radicals during such prolonged physical activity. Dr. Cooper theorized that the low-density lipoprotein cholesterol or LDL-C (bad cholesterol) binds with the free radicals in the coronary arteries and produces something called "foam cells," an atheroma, which, he deduced, unnoticeably congested Jim Fixx's arteries.

And it only makes sense that, since we are dealing with a stress—just like sunlight—chronic, gross overtraining can inordinately tax the overall physiologic system and possibly result in a breakdown where there might be a weak link, like the lymphatic and endocrine systems or, in the case of the vascular system, an inflammation that could result in very serious state of health.

The research behind the negative aspects of overtraining is overwhelming and it continues to build up enormous sums of evidence showing why one should avoid over-exercise. Clearly there is some major correlation between physical activity and life expectancy...just not as we traditionally believe.

Exercise is necessitated by the nature of man in order for him to live as long and as strong as possible...but by our physiologic nature, by our *specific* design, we are not meant to be tirelessly active. Aerobics, cardio, endurance running, call it what you will, are against human nature and destructive. Do the names Euchidas or Pheidippides sound familiar? Both men are of legend with their respective run of an ultramarathon—though not for health benefits—and both finished the race by dropping dead. And yet, instead of detouring people from the detriment of long distant running, there are "marathons" held all over the place (Marathon being the location in Greece where Pheidippides ran to Athens) and ultra-marathons, like the International Spartathlon race, that span the same supposed length of Pheidippides' run to death. What is more, there are countless examples of such an ultimate result, directly caused by such over-exercise.

Aerobics are worse than useless…worse because they offer no potential benefits of exercise, but still hold all of the negatives. In order for any activity to show any signs of progress, you must perform that activity for a greater amount of time or intensity…one or the other, never both. The problem with aerobics…well, one of many…is that in order to continue to get results you have to increase the duration of the activity, thus resulting in you soon reaching a point where you are overtraining. My advice to anyone reading this who still insists on performing aerobics—i.e. calisthenics, marathon running, or any "endurance" activity—for health benefits is…wakeup! Only a fool would continue to put their body in danger for no productive reason, and you are a fool if you are one of them….

Harsh words? Hey, no one every said that the truth is pretty…but don't blame me if you are a fool…I didn't make you one.

142 *Logical H.I.T.*

Let me put is this way, I would not want to be a marathon runner 10, 000 years ago trying to kill a deer for food that is the difference between life and death, when I could have the physical strength to kill that deer with my bare hands if I was weaponless and had to protect myself from predators ever lurking around me. And believe me, when you are faced with the alternative of you and your family starving, you will do what you can to get food...and the stronger you were the better your chances of eating were.

Not possible you say? Well many individuals have proven otherwise, my great uncle was one of them...a man whose strength saved many lives by carrying panic-stricken construction workers off steel beams towering hundreds of feet in the air, who also had the strength to punch a deer to death when his gun jammed.

So, when you find yourself in the possession of a larger and stronger body, you will be in a position that will allow you a better chance of survival...a state that seems to be favored in nature over that of the excessively active aerobics cult.

6

The Haircut Study

Recovery & Intensity: Conception and Thesis

I initiated this study in early 2008 for the simplistic, yet prolific, query of, what is the minimum amount of volume & frequency of exercise required in order to elicit the greatest gains in muscular strength and size possible. The ingenious works of Mike Mentzer and Doug McGuff seeded this inquiry and it was stimulated by the reasoning mind of John Little.

The most productive, and ultimately, correct component of optimum bodybuilding progress is the established fact that it is least amount of exercise that is required to stimulate the body's growth mechanism into motion that is all that is required. Upon intellectual digesting such a logical fact of human physiology, I questioned in what way this is structured within proper training practices. Mike Mentzer insistently stated that you would interrupt your recovery process, thus your muscle growth, by performing anymore more sets and/ or greater frequency of workouts than the least amount required, as you would disturb or throw a preverbal wrench in the growth mechanism of the body. When I heard this, I immediately concluded that this statement held a deeper meaning and that it was the key in discovering the most productive method to conduct one's training efforts in order to produce the greatest muscular gains possible—why not just perform one set. Why do I postulate that one set of one high intensity exercise is all that is physiologically required when individuals obtain phenomenal growth by performing 2 to 5 exercises in a workout of one set each exercise? This question flourished into the inquisition to discover the truth.

Physiologically, the body's biochemical reserves deplete upon the imposition of a stress or stresses imposed upon it. Why the investigation of only one set? It is because a second set is not a mere liner increase of one to two in the depletion of your body's adaptive energies, but a 100 percent increase in the amount of exercise, thus a doubling of the deficit you have imposed on your body's limited reserve of resources. However, a conjectural opposition would state, "What if a second set of that exercise stimulated a little more growth?" This however is nullified by the fact that, even if a second set did stimulated 100 percent more growth, the benefit would be negated by the mere fact that you have doubled the debt in your body's *limited* adaptive energies and, in most cases, individuals do not stimulate 100 percent more muscle growth. Therefore, there is impedance, a net loss, of the maximal gains that first set could have, should have, yielded.

The importance of only performing the least amount of exercise necessary to stimulate muscle growth is pointed out in the following explanation. When you perform only one set to momentary muscular failure, you have thus stimulated the body's growth mechanism into motion, but have also consumed the least amount of adaptive resources possible while still stimulating growth. Having much more resources leftover to facility the greatest growth possible, as long as you do not disturb the body in the process with more exercise. Ideally, you could stimulate muscle growth with no sets, upon which you would deplete none of your body's adaptive reserves. Furthermore, in doing so, with no sacrifice of your body's energy reserves all your adaptive energy would be forwarded towards muscle growth instead of recovering. As a result, you would grow so damn fast that it would stagger the imagination.

This fact confirmed in me an answer beneath the shroud of tradition. Others have reached the same conclusion and, in doing so, cultivated a moral value in finding the scientifically required quantity of training volume and frequency. However, all of them went by the means of progressively doing less than before. Where upon reaching a point where results exceeded their expectations they stop: morally gratified. I had started obscure of tradition and concretized mentally the certainty that it is the least amount required—in this case, one set—which is all that is economically necessary.

As a result, on this premise I began a study, having 7 individuals perform only one set a workout! Not one set per exercise, which is the commonplace of most HIT enthusiast, but merely one set in the fashion that Mike later in his personal training career dabbled with before his death. I had sought for the truth at the most logical position of search: the beginning or the nadir of the account. The founding pillar of this premise stands on the factor that post-stimulation recovery is equally as important as the stimulus itself. Acknowledging this, the study group began training once every one to two weeks, and then later increased to once every three to even four weeks in some cases. As a measure of efficiency, I had a control group training on Mike Mentzer's consolidation routine that consists of one weekly training session of two exercises. This routine has already been empirically proven as one of the most, if not the most, productive training routines ever formulated.

The Research

Prior to the initiation of this study I personally weighed and measured the calves, thighs, hips, waist, chest, shoulders, and upper arms of all of the research subjects. Furthermore I analyzed the subcutaneous body fat of the subjects with a clinically approved skin fold caliper. Reaching the eight-week mark, I tested and calculated their up to date results. Assessing the strength gain of the control-training group, I found that their average strength gain was 23 percent. The group's body fat decreased an average of 2.4 percent and their average muscular gain was 5.2lbs.

When I tested the individuals of the study's attention, I found that their average strength gain was 41 percent! Their average fat loss was 2.1 percent, but when assessing their average muscular gain I was absolutely baffled by the astonishing fact that one individual (Samantha Diller), a female volunteer, gained an unimaginable 17 lbs of muscle in only five workouts! The average muscle gain for the study group was 9.5lbs!

One factor that I want to state now so there are

no misinterpretations is that no volunteers were made to change their diets, with food consumption under their own free will and none of them were instructed to perform any aerobics. The only thing I personally implemented in their supplementary consumption was packets of ordinary table sugar, used after a high intensity set of exercise in order to bring the volunteers back to their baseline of physical functional ability as quickly as possible.

Findings in the third quarter of the study had shown that a training frequency of once every three to four weeks—for a continuously scheduled regime—has allowed the volunteers to still progress in strength, but at a much slower rate than they were at a 1 to 2 week interval. I had begun drawing a few conclusions from this research so far, with one leading into a further hypothesis. First of all, I am realizing that individuals that train at very low volumes of sets *vastly* reduce the length of needed recovery time; even one set more—the performance of two or three sets—I found can lower the progress of some individuals in the next workout one week later with intermediate to advance subjects.

During this study, I also performed some complementary sub-studies where I subjected individuals that perform one set workouts once every two weeks to a few advance high intensity training techniques. Astonishingly I found that with frequent usage of advanced high intensity training techniques, a few individuals, whose progress was averaging a 20 to 40 pound jump in leg press and a 10 to 20 pound increase in upper body movements dropped approximately 45 percent by their next workout, only being moderate increases in strength.

Seeing this dramatic decrease in progress has confirmed my assumption that training intensity can be toxic or counter productive beyond momentary muscular failure (positive muscular failure), without hyper cautious regulation of the frequency and volume of the workout.

One hypothesis that I wish to pursue in a later study is that, if an individual stays on a frequency of once every three weeks, would their annual net gain come to a greater total than a standard commonly practiced H.I.T routine? This would be a very interesting topic to research, as I have based it on the model of a trainee becoming very sensitive to high intensity training as they become more advanced. They will eventually become in need of a lower training frequency merely to catch up with the considerable inroad that they have induced, not to mention produce a muscular surplus.

Coming to the conclusion of this study, with the study group training once every three to four weeks, has shown some very dramatic results and I have begun drawing three conclusions. One, the individuals, in a number of cases, became slightly to extremely nauseous due to the build-up of metabolic by-products, due to, what I believe, was a deconditioning of their cardiovascular efficiency. Two, the strength fell in some individuals and only increased small increments in others; this result could be due to previous and the next conclusion. Third, in almost all cases, the motivational level of all volunteers dropped after not training for three weeks.

One of the major conclusions that I am seeing is that the overall debt in biochemical resources determines the required frequency of one's workouts. Since I reduced the volume of the entire research group's workouts so dramatically, the total physiologic deficit was not severe enough to warrant an infrequency of once every three weeks, at least not at their current level of strength. This study demonstrates that the adding of one set is not merely a sequential increase in the volume of the workout; it is a 100 percent increase in the volume of the workout and makes that much more of a drain on your limited reserve resources. Every high intensity set consumes an enormous quantity of resources (depending on the size and number of muscles used).

In addition to the study group, I had one individual in the research group who trained once every 3 to 4 weeks with two to three sets per workout. This individual was, in fact, progressing tremendously (Rob Cunningham), but this individual also was performing athletic activities that most likely contributed to his zealous motivation to train hard.

At the end of the study, the individuals in the study group had only two weeks respite, due to academic responsibilities. After the initial response and conclusions drawn from the previous results of little or retrogressive results, I pre-concluded that their results would be unchanged or even negatively changed. During the final body composition and strength test, I was incredulous! Their body fat had decreased and they gained weight. Their measurements showed increases in all major musculatures and decreases in waist and slightly hip girth.

The strength test would be the deciding factor in this amazement—maybe they were just coming down from a higher level of muscle gain. The volunteers were placed into the machines and were quite enthusiastic. Out of curiosity, I jumped the weight 10 to 20 pounds from their previous bests, before the extreme infrequencies. And in all cases their strength increased...dramatically!

They were extraordinarily focused and performed in a slower fashion than they did in their first initial strength test with many more repetitions—one individual lifting 70 percent more weight than her initial strength test and performing 35 more repetitions. Then something came to me as I was being stupefied by these results: their metabolic conditioning. The metabolic systems of the body, including the ever-popular aerobic system, require insignificant amounts of biochemical material to adapt and perform with higher levels of efficiency than muscle tissue, of which, requires huge amounts of raw material for hypertrophy. After only a two week respite their metabolic systems had up regulated substantially faster than their muscular tissue. This, of which, has demonstrated to me and the volunteers of the study how efficiently proper high intensity training improves the overall functional ability of the body.

The Results

<u>Control Group Body Compositions</u>

Jordan Nicolson	**02/04/2008**	**06/03/2008**
Body Fat	16%	10.2% [-5.8]
Weight / lean	164.5lbs [138lbs]	172lbs [155lbs]
Jill Brown	**02/04/2008**	**06/03/2008**
Body Fat	23.5%	19.84% [-3.66]
Weight / lean	119lbs [91lbs]	119lbs [96lbs]
Brian Mills	**02/04/2008**	**06/06/2008**
Body Fat	10.7%	5.87% [-4.83]
Weight / lean	143lbs [128lbs]	140.5lbs [133lbs]
Billy Mino	**02/04/2008**	**06/06/2008**
Body Fat	15.12%	8.03% [-7.09]
Weight / lean	149lbs [127lbs]	150lbs [138]
Mitchell Smith	**02/05/2008**	**06/04/2008**
Body Fat	16.4%	11.65% [-4.75]
Weight / lean	159lbs [133lbs]	161lbs [143lbs]
Jason Campbell	**02/05/2008**	**06/04/2008**
Body Fat	10.3%	8.25% [-2.05]
Weight / lean	146lbs [132lbs]	154lbs [142lbs]

Totals & Averages

Total weight gained	16lbs
Total fat loss	40.32lbs
Total muscle gain	58lbs
Average muscle gain	9.67lbs
Average fat loss	6.72lbs
Most muscle gained	17lbs
Most fat lost	10.63lbs

Number of Workouts

Jordan Nicolson	#16
Jill Brown	#16
Brian Mills	#13
Billy Mino	#11
Jason Campbell	#15
Mitchell Smith	#15

Study Group Body Compositions

Erica Wright	**02/03/2008**	**06/04/2008**
Body Fat	26.95%	21.1% [-5.85]
Weight / lean	135.5lbs [99lbs]	144lbs [114lbs]
Sarah Alexander	**02/03/2008**	**06/02/2008**
Body Fat	21.72%	17.9% [-3.82]
Weight / lean	116.5lbs [92lbs]	123lbs [101lbs]
Samantha Diller	**02/02/2008**	**06/02/2008**
Body Fat	27.5%	22.9% [-4.6]
Weight / lean	150lbs [108lbs]	163lbs [126lbs]
Jordan McMullen	**02/02/2008**	**06/02/2008**
Body Fat	12.8%	8.36% [-4.44]
Weight / lean	154lbs [135lbs]	156lbs [143lbs]
Micah Simmons	**02/06/2008**	**06/03/2008**
Body Fat	13.5%	8.75% [-4.75]
Weight / lean	192lbs [167lbs]	192lbs [176lbs]
Dustin Manley	**02/05/2008**	**06/06/2008**
Body Fat	14.6%	8.97% [-5.63]
Weight / lean	140lbs [120lbs]	141.5lbs [129lbs]
Rob Cunningham	**04/24/2008**	**06/06/2008**
Body Fat	20.38%	14.31% [-6.07]
Weight / lean	196.5lbs [157lbs]	207lbs [178lbs]

Totals & Averages

Total weight gained	41.5lbs
Total fat loss	47.2lbs
Total muscle gain	89lbs
Average muscle gain	12.7lbs
Average fat loss	6.74lbs
Most muscle gained	21lbs
Most fat lost	10.43lbs

Number of Workouts

Erica Wright	#10
Jordan McMullen	#10
Samantha Diller	#10
Sarah Alexander	#8
Micah Simmons	#7
Dustin Manley	#7
Rob Cunningham	#4

Conclusions

Throughout this study I have learned an extraordinary amount about the effects of high intensity training on the human body. I have found some techniques that improved the results of muscle growth and discovered some of the important factors of recovery ability brought forth with an immense physiologic stimulus:

• It seems that the performance of higher intensity protocols, such as, rest pause, infitonic training, Omni contraction and hyper repetitions can become considerably counterproductive in concert with the customary recovery period ascribed to regular high intensity programs. This fact was quite unexpected with some of the genetically gifted individuals, as they, being able to tolerate much greater quantities of exercise, were still being negatively affected when performing advanced techniques continuously in their training program. A logical answer to this is that, yes they are able to recover faster and do have a much deeper reserve of adaptation energy from which to draw upon. However, these individuals are able to become stronger at a staggeringly greater rate than the individuals average to lesser genetic potential. Because of this, they are able to quickly overwhelm the recovery margins of their body.

The body's adaptation energy reserves do have the capacity to increase, but not even close to the same rate as the muscle's strength. The muscles, clearly, have the capacity to increase there draining capability by approximately 300 percent, while the body's adaptation reserves only have the capacity for an approximate 50 percent increase, but more like 25 percent in many cases. As a result, when performing any advance techniques that further deepen the drain of your body's adaptive energies you run the risk of lessening your body's ability to reap the most from what the workout stimulated, for the mere act of replenishing the extensive deficit of the workout.

• Every set performed in a workout demands an extraordinary amount of the body's biochemical resources. Findings from the study demonstrably showed that even one set could require two weeks to recover from and obtain the maximal potential of the muscle growth stimulated in some cases.

• Performing exercises in a slower manner, ranging on a repetition speed of 2-4 on the positive and negative aspect of the lift and 1-2 seconds in the fully contracted position showed to be much more productive than the employment of faster repetition cadences. This was attributed to the fact that the muscle was loaded under a significant tension the entire set and were not allowed to obtain any unloading respite for recovering its lower order motor units, as would be the case with momentum's interlude. However, performing a very slow styled cadence in the barbell squat and deadlift impaired the breathing ability of the participants. This is attributed to having an increase in pressure on the abdominal and thoracic cavities in the bottom position. I found that the main concern with the deadlift and the squat should be to focus on exercising control over counting your cadence. The main issue is to prevent momentum from coming into the exercise, so perform the squat and the deadlift deliberately and under full muscular control.

• In almost every case, with one or two highly motivated exceptions, the volunteers that were told to take a three to four week respite noted that their motivation for working out dropped substantially after two weeks and their results were less than they were with once every one to two weeks. However, this is not the rule, for example, John Little has made mention of one of his phone consultation clients working out once every six weeks performing merely one set and gaining 18 pounds of muscle in 8 months. Though this individual is an advanced trainee, requiring a prolonged period of rest between workouts, he still possesses the vital motivation and a comprehension of his value to be gained from intense, very brief and, in his case, extremely infrequent exercise.

• Workouts containing a maximum of three exercises were extraordinarily draining among a few of the volunteers in the control group. With some, I had no choice but to reduce their workouts to two exercises. This further confirmed my conviction of a non-need of more than two-three exercise a workout for most individuals.

• The greatest fact I learned from this study was intensity's role in the equation of proper exercise. A proper workout can be analyzed like an algebraic equation, with three interrelated variables: Frequency, Volume and Intensity. Now, the identities and causalities of volume and frequency were already very much established years ago. However, the role of intensity was incomplete. Mike Mentzer was the one who started to reach this conclusion and began to understand intensity's delicate role in the pursuit of the greatest achievable progress.

High intensity is required for muscle growth, just as a *specific* volume of sets and frequency is required. But it too can be carried to extremes just like volume and frequency. This study became not only a search to find the optimal volume and frequency, but intensity as well. What is needed in terms of intensity is appropriately identified in the same manner as its two adjoining aspects: it is the least amount required to produce the desired result that is optimal. And since the only measurable level of productive intensity is 100 percent momentary muscular failure in the positive advancement of an exercise, it is possible that positive failure is optimal.

(Note: though this study demonstrated fantastic results from brief, infrequent and intense exercise I still remain unsatisfied due to the lack of a greater pool of subjects to test...additionally, I hoped to have a more controlled environment for which to train the subjects and more productive tools for which to test and train them. But as of now, I am in the process of, or already have obtained, since the conclusion of this experiment, more productive tools; a controlled training environment, allowing no outside disturbances; tools capable of measuring and recording the experiment in a manner that removes all doubt as to the validity of the results, including video recordings of each an every workout; and finally, a much larger pool of subjects with a much greater age range. The results of said experiment—multiple actually, which will vary from frequency needs to the productivity of intensification protocols when weighed against one another—will expectedly be available in a future book or online.)

Part III
Theory into Praxis

"If NASA can send a man to the moon and return him safely each time—an enormously complex task requiring the application of theoretical knowledge from intellectual disciplines such as mathematics, physics, computer technology, medicine, rocket science, etc.—we should be able to succeed with every one of our missions to the gym here on earth. That should be a cakewalk instead of a moonwalk!?

Mike Mentzer, Bodybuilder, Philosopher and Trainer

"Today's scientists have substituted mathematics for experiments, and they wander off through equation after equation, and eventually build a structure which has no relation to reality."

Nikola Tesla, Inventor and Engineer

7

Key Knowledge of an Intelligent Bodybuilder

In order for you to bring forth the most from your training efforts, there are a few prerequisites that need to be grasped first. I have condensed the experiences of my training career with my clients, my own training and my extensive research into a set of training prerequisite guidelines that must be grasped before you setoff on your high intensity program.

Muscle Fiber Type Continued...

Previously I touched upon the role of muscle fiber type in muscular size/strength potential: slow twitch fibers having lower size/strength potential, but with great endurance; contrasted with fast twitch fibers having large size/strength potential, but low endurance; with intermediate fibers somewhere in the middle. However, what I did not discuss was how having a predominance of one or the other could significantly alter your training needs. To begin explaining the significance of muscle fiber type I will start with a brief account of my own experience with the significance of muscle fiber predominance in my training.

After the experiment I conducted with super high volume training, which is mentioned in chapter 5, I started on a typical high intensity three-way split routine: training once every seven days, performing four to five exercises, one set each, with a repetition range of 8-15 for upper body exercises and 12-20 for lower body exercises. But since I was preoccupied with the Haircut study, school, my own personal research and working at Nautilus North five days a week, I was completely imperturbable as far as my training was concerned...at the time. Looking back at my training charts after a number of months, however, regaled me with something that I didn't take-in so warmly at the time as I do now—which is usually the case when someone discovers that they have been wasting countless hours of effort to get nowhere. My progress was, to put it frankly, horrible. I was so caught up in the astounding progress of the volunteers in the Haircut study and the clientele at Nautilus North that I was blind to the fact that my progress left something to be desired.

In an effort to rectify my lack of progress, I started jumping from one protocol to another: rest-pause, partial reps, SuperSlow, forced reps, max contraction and almost any other you can think of. But alas, I was still barely able to make the scale display positive results... and my training charts were not much better in terms of progress. Nevertheless, I knew that the theory of high intensity training was the one and only correct theory of bodybuilding exercise—I had seen far too much evidence to prove otherwise, moreover, I had utilized a crude version of HIT before my little experiment and grew considerably—, yet I still could not help but feel a little frustrated. Nevertheless, I did not dismiss high intensity training out of hand because of frustration—though I have not been the smartest person in the world at times, when

I encounter such seemingly self-evident facts of reality that are apparent to a dead fish, I usually take notice of the fact that they have some undeniable value.

After a thorough period of literature wondering, I decided to reread and re-reread the works of Mike Mentzer and Arthur Jones. And it was when I turned to Heavy Duty II, on page 85, that I became excited by something that had little to no meaning to me the last time I encountered it, but was the most important turning point of my thinking the second time through—which is why I suggested in the opening of this book that you reread and re-reread it…you never know, something just might be meaningless to you at one point, but worth the world to you at another.

What caused such excitement in me was a problem that Mike Mentzer faced with one client, Racy Chatterji. In this case, it seemed that, no matter what Mike did, Racy would not grow bigger or stronger. However, possessing intellectual certainty, Mike knew that the theory of high intensity training was correct, but knew that there was something decidedly wrong, not with the theory, but with his application of it.

After scaling back Racy's training volume and frequency significantly, and repeatedly, Racy started to grow. It was with much deliberation and study that Mike Mentzer was able to grasp that, just as all human physical characteristics are expressed on a broad continuum, with midgets and medical morons on one extreme and geniuses and eight-foot giants on the other, Racy was obviously, to put it candidly, a midget or moron in the case of his recovery ability and growth potential. (Racy, being an intelligent and rational individual, found much humor in Mike's straightforward analogy of liking his recovery ability and growth potential to that of the stature of a midget.)

So did the pleasure in this reexamination come from discovering that I was midget or moron of recovery ability and muscle growth—absolutely not! The fact of the matter was that *I was not focusing on my genetic predisposition*; I was applying the physiologic parameters of the usual to the physiologic parameters of what deviated from the usual, the unusual. The truth is that I am on the other extreme of that continuum…nevertheless, that has also hindered me tremendously in my high intensity training from when I picked it up again after my high volume experiment—an experiment that, unknowingly, cloaked me in many fallacies and obscurities.

But as someone once said…"A wise man can see more from the bottom of a well than a fool can from a mountain top." And in this case, I was, without doubt, at the bottom of well, but wise or not, I was determined to discover why…why did it seem as if all I was doing was taking one step forward and two steps back?

While studying genetics far more painstakingly than any time before, it wasn't until I read through *My First Half-Century in the Iron Game* by Arthur Jones that I began to grasp my disposition. Muscle fiber type predominance, it appeared, can alter one's training needs far more than I ever thought. In one case, Arthur Jones was introduced to an individual who could bench press 605 pounds in perfect form. Quite impressed with this individual, Arthur began contemplating his possibilities if he was trained correctly. So, knowing that you should not use your maximum poundage when trying to increase strength, Arthur gave this individual 480 pounds and asked him to perform as many repetitions as possible.

However, Arthur was astonished when this individual

was only able to perform three repetitions, when he expected this individual to perform ten to eleven repetitions. But, lacking the knowledge that was to come from future years of research with thousands of individuals utilizing the only machines that can accurately measure strength (MedX), Arthur formed the poor opinion that this individual was just not trying, while, unbeknownst to him, this individual had been giving it his all. This particular individual possessed an unusually high percentage of fast twitch fibers in the musculature that is utilized in the bench press movement, which allowed him to lift significant poundage, but hindered him as far as muscular endurance was concerned.

In a more relevant case to bodybuilding history buffs, when Arthur Jones was testing Casey Viator on a bench press machine that displayed his force output and required him to perform as many repetitions as possible, with the machine making every repetition maximal, Casey was only able to perform eight repetitions. After every successive repetition, Casey's strength drastically declined until, on his eighth repetition, he was *ninety-two* percent weaker than his fresh strength. But on the ninth repetition, Casey was literally producing *zero* positive output force, no matter how hard he tried. Having failed to understand it at the time, Arthur wished to demonstrate such astounding results to a group of scientists for their benefit, if not his. This time Casey was stationed in a leg press version of this machine and was asked to perform as many repetitions as possible.

While Arthur was certain that he would have Casey demonstrate the same result to the scientists as the one that was seen on the bench press version of that machine, Arthur was astonished when, after more than thirty repetitions Casey showed almost no slightest sign of fatigue. It was after a period of research and experimentation that Arthur concluded that Casey possessed an unusually high percentage of fast twitch fibers in the musculature that is utilized in the bench press, but an equally unusual percentage of slow twitch fibers in the musculature of his thighs and hips. With this and other research, Arthur found that individuals with unusually high percentages of fast twitch fibers would be better off performing lower repetitions ranging from three to six, but that they *require* much less frequency of exercise due to their poor recovery speed; slow twitch subjects do better with higher repetitions ranging from fifteen to twenty and are capable of, but are better off not, training more often than average individuals; and finally, that the majority of individuals, who are a "usual" mixture, are better off with six to twelve repetitions.

Breakthrough—Was this it? Was this the key of illumination that I had lost, preventing me from unlocking the capabilities of my physiology? After some deeper contemplation of my training past before the experiment, though volumous compared to sane standards, was intense, with every set carried to failure (though I did not take every working set to failure out of the knowledge that it was required by the nature of human physiology, I trained to failure because I always had the mindset that if you truly want something you have to give it everything you've got). However, remembering the actually details of my training I came to realize that my repetitions were, in general, fairly low, ranging from four to eight. With this, I began to experiment and ultimately I found that most of my muscles are constituted of an unusually high percentage of fast twitch fibers. With this, I realized that my time under load on my exercises, the number of repetitions, were far too high, thus, limiting my true potential of utilizing a productive resistance. Where even with Max Contraction and rest-pause, I was performing these protocols in the second stage of a pre-exhaust cycle, thus, already having weakened my predominate musculature to a dramatic degree, I was merely kicking myself in the ass instead of doing any good.

Now while this was only one of a list of mistakes that I made at the time, though definitely not as detrimental as others that I will get to later, it did hold me back from even greater results down the road.

The ideal weight to use for the purpose of increasing muscular size and strength is approximately eighty to seventy-five percent of your maximum fresh strength. And when you have a high percentage of fast twitch fibers, you are usually capable of only performing three to six repetitions. In my case, my average rep range is approximately four to eight in most movements.

For that reason, after a few months on the recommended rep ranges presented in the next chapter, if you find that after applying all of the principles correctly, allowing adequate recovery time and training to momentary muscular failure, you are not able to increase the number of repetitions you can perform to the high end of the prescribed rep range or that you can easily increase your number of repetitions the next workout but can only increase the weight utilized on that rep scheme very infrequently, you may have a high predominance of either fast or slow twitch fibers. At that point, you may want to perform a strength test in which you attempt to find your one repetition maximum on each exercise, performed in a *very* strict and controlled manner, four seconds up, if there is tension in the fully contracted position hold for two seconds, and lower in four seconds. (Attempting a maximal repetition with carelessness and with no focus on lifting against the resistance in proper form, just throwing it, only assures that you are subjecting your joints and connective tissues to dangerous levels of impact force.) Besides making sure you have one or more strong spotters to make sure that you are not overwhelmed when trying to find your maximum weight that you can handle for one repetition, make sure that you spend adequate time warming up prior—unlike multiple repetition sets, a single maximum effort lift does not possess a built-in warm-up that makes sure that the joints and muscles acquire ample blood flood and warmth prior to a maximal effort.

Once you find your one rep max, your next workout use eighty to seventy-five percent of your maximum and performing as many repetitions as possible in good form. If you find that you fail within one of the ranges described above (3-6 fast, 8-12 usual, 15-20 slow twitch), you are highly apt to being that subject type in those muscles. Although this method is crude and not perfectly accurate, it will give you a starting point. Once figuring out your general types and rep ranges in each exercise, you can experiment with repetition ranges that come close to your muscles' capabilities. However, I do not recommend that you perform this test on either the squat or the deadlift, for two reasons. First of all, in both cases, you are dealing with the delicate articulation of the lumbar spine, performing a single maximal lift can inordinately stress the structural integrity of the lumbar region, so a sub-maximal workout is far safer. Secondly, since performing the squat and the deadlift with a maximal weight requires a great deal of skill, you are susceptible to causing harm because of poor form.

These two exercises should never be performed in a maximal, signal rep fashion unless you are training for a powerlifting competition. Instead of performing this strength test to find you more profitable rep range, you will have to do some experimentation with rep ranges and monitor your progress as you alter the range...but never go below six repetitions on either exercise. You will eventually become very strong, by any standard, on this routine, so performing low rep, near maximal lifts will become very risky. However, as of yet, I have not seen an individual that does not benefit from repetition ranging from 12 to 20 on the squat or 8 to 15 on the deadlift. Though they may be "high" repetition sets, which will require you to lower the weight, they will in no way be easier...if done right, these will be the most intense physically and emotionally demanding exercises of your life. The range is high because a 4-2-4 cadence is often impractical and results in an inadequate time under load with the 6-10 range prescribed for other exercises.

For the majority of individuals utilizing the program described in this book, the prescribed range of repetitions are excellent in terms of inroading and overloading the average individual's musculature and producing tremendous results. Yet there are still exceptional individuals out there who would be better off performing either more or less repetitions in order to adequately inroad their muscles and overloading them with a sufficient weight. Having a fast twitch subject inroad his quadriceps to a point where they are incapable of lifting a 160 pound resistance, when they are capable of contracting against a 250 pound resistance for six repetitions, is inroading his quadriceps muscles to such an undesirable extent that it almost defies sanity. And the same thing applies when you try to productively inroad a slow twitch predominate muscle by forcing it to contract against nearly all the weight it can handle for one repetition when it requires in excess of fifteen such repetitions to actually recruit and fatigue all available fibers.

Muscle growth is a multifactorial process that requires a proper balance of all factors that contribute the process. Overindulgence of one factor could, and will eventually, adversely affect the whole process: inroad taken too far will negatively affect the individual's recovery time and the amount of resistance that can be utilized (unless you are performing negative-only type of exercise, in which case you will quickly lead to overtraining if not hyper-cautious); too much weight will not allow for a beneficial inroad or the stimulation of productive metabolic adaptations, etc. Perfect balance of these factors is a relative term: who is the individual training, how long has he been training for and does he have any injuries, past or present? All such factors that can influence their needed balance. But all things being equal (with no injuries that hinder performance, in addition to having been training for a period of time that has allowed their body the chance to hypertrophy any dormant fast twitch fibers that atrophy quickly without proper stimulation—resulting in a false impression of slow twitch predominance, when it is only because the fast twitch fibers have been allowed to atrophy to a point that they take on some slow twitch characteristics), all things being equal, it is an individual's muscle fiber profile that seems to ultimately dictate this ratio.

Internal Muscular Friction

Earlier I touched upon the subject of internal muscular friction, of which, prevents you from expressing your true strength in the positive aspect of any lift, is null and void in the static or holding of the weight in any position throughout a given range of motion, and adds to your strength in the lowering aspect of a lift. But why is this... and what import does it have in your training?

In order to comprehend such a simple, yet seemingly complex, fact we will need to grasp some very basic laws of physics, in particular, the laws of motion. And, in doing so, we are introduced to a man named Isaac Newton.

Isaac Newton, probably one of the greatest minds in the history of mankind, compiled the three fundamental laws of motion in his work *Philosophiæ Naturalis Principia Mathematica,* in 1687. Laws that are universal, they apply to everything, which includes muscles.

Newton's first law: the law of inertia—Simply put, Newton's first law of motion states "*a body persists its state of rest or of uniform motion unless acted upon by an external unbalanced force*". Meaning, an entity with mass will not move unless it is acted upon by a great enough force that can overcome its inertia (inertia being an objects resistance to changes in its state of motion). This means for the bodybuilder, that in order for you to positively lift a barbell weighing 100 pounds vertically you must initial produce an *output* force that is more than 100 pounds to accelerate the barbell into an upward direction. Then once you have initiated movement, overcoming inertia, you must reduce your output force to *exactly* 100 pounds in order to maintain a constant velocity. Once you have overcome inertia you must to reduce your *output* force to a level equal to the opposing force of the barbell, if not, you will continue to accelerate.

However, if you reduce your output force to 99 pounds, the barbell will begin to deaccelerate until it stops progressive movement, at which point, if you increased your output force back to 100 pounds, you would hold that barbell statically or what is called isometrically. Yet, if you produced one pound more output force the barbell would rise, one pound less and it would begin to descend. If you were to reduce your output force, so as to allow the barbell to initiate a descending motion, once the barbell begins to descend you would produce 100 pounds of output force again to prevent it from accelerating downward....But can this be right?

Of course it is. Inertia is an entity's resistance to *changes* in its state of motion. Once you have overcome the initial resistance of inertia, all you have to do in order to persist in that state of motion is overcome outside forces that oppose you...namely gravity in this case, of which, acts in a consistent and fixed manner. All of which summates into the fact that, in order for you to perform an exercise in a safe and productive manner, you must accelerate the resistance just enough to move it in the desired direction, then reduce you output force just enough to maintain a constant velocity until you need to increase or decrease your force output for the next phase of the exercise.

If you do not believe me, go and buy a spring scale like the ones used at your local grocery store, and try this little experiment. Attach a five pound weight to the end of the scale, look at the scale and observe the reading of five pounds, then move the weight at a slow and constant speed upwards. Doing so, you will notice that the scale reads only a slight increase in weight, but then quickly returns to that five pound measurement as long as you keep that constant velocity. Then when you smoothly reverse that motion into a constant downward velocity, you will see that the scale briefly reads a measurement less than five pounds, but then returns to five pounds. What you are observing is the fact that, as long as the velocity is constant, there is only a minor differential in the force you are exerting and, thus, only a small change in the force you are exposing your joints and soft tissues to the moment you change the weight's direction of movement.

Newton's second law—When you are lifting against a resistance, whether it is a barbell or the moment arm of a machine connected to a weight stack, you are lifting against gravity. If you take a barbell into outer space where there is no gravity, its *mass* remains the same, constant, unvarying… but it has no *weight*. Weight is a relative term, one that is expressed by a gravitational pull or acceleration action upon something in concert with a force opposing that acceleration. Your weight or *downward force* that you read on your scale when you step on it in the morning is the result of the earth's gravitational pull accelerating your mass 9.81 m/s^2 into the ground with the scale opposing your downward acceleration with equal and opposite force.

Newton's second law of motion states, "*Force equals mass times by acceleration.*" This, in terms of your training, means that rapidly accelerating the weight in either direction subjects your joints to much greater impact force that *only* serves to harm you, with absolutely *nothing* in the way of benefit.

Although it is impossible to perform productive exercise without exposing your muscles and connective tissues to a meaningful force, an abrupt dramatic escalation in the force you subject your body to will most likely have the potential of exceeding the structural strength of your connective tissues. For example, let's say that the structural strength of your connective tissues were 100 pounds, which means that anything over 100 pounds will compromise their structural integrity and they will rupture. In utilizing a 75 pound resistance, moving in a slow and deliberate manner, you are well within your connective tissue's acceptable parameters with only insignificant oscillations in the force you are exposing your tissues to, while still exposing your muscles and connective tissue to a meaningful enough load that will cause them to enlarge upon their physiologic margins—thus becoming stronger. Now let's say that you use that same 75 pound resistance, but, instead of slowly lifting it, you rapidly accelerate it upwards and then let it drop down during the negative. In this latter scenario, you have now produced such tremendous impact force that it will unquestionably exceed 100 pounds in the lifting phase of the movement…but even more so if you drop the weight instead of slowly lowering it. Dropping a 75 pound barbell, allowing gravity to accelerate it downwards, can produce an impact force in excess of 350 pounds on the muscle, connective tissues and the joint when they are forced to catch the accelerating weight in the full-extended position, resulting in multiple hundreds percent more force being imposed on your soft tissues… and this *will* do nothing in the way of benefit…it is, however, an extremely productive, and quick, manner to destroy your joints, I can guarantee that much.

The lesson of this little story is that, in order for exercise to be productive and safe, it must be of *high* intensity...but *low* force. Now do not be dissuaded by the illogical claims that any higher force equals better growth stimulation—only a dangerous fool tries to live by such a code of bodybuilding conduct. Yes you require force acting on the tissues you wish to stimulate into development, and that force *must* be meaningful enough to get the attention of the body, but a reckless loading of these tissues with fluctuations between severe impact force trauma and the unloading weightless effect of momentum is nothing less than the apex of insanity.

The most effective manner to train with the intention of increasing muscular size and strength is to use *sub-*maximal weights that allow you to inroad or bring down your maximal strength to the point where that chosen weight *becomes* maximal. Doing this you avoid compromising the structural integrity of your connective tissues, yet still expose them to a significant enough load that will give them all of the incentive required for them to increase their structural strength.

Newton's third law: law of reciprocal actions—Now, the highlight of the three laws of motion, Newton's third law of motion states, "*To every action there is always an equal and opposite reaction.*" However, for our needs, this can also be presented as, *everything with both mass and motion has friction...*including muscle.

While discussing the first law of motion I made the statement that you were to lift a 100 pound weight vertically at a constant velocity, with absolutely no acceleration, you would require 100 pounds of *output* force to maintain that velocity. Then I said that holding the weight would also require you to produce 100 pounds of output force, next I stated that if you were to lower that weight at a constant velocity you would need to produce 100 pounds of output force. But here is the issue…why is it harder to lift a weight than it is to hold it in any one position? Moreover, why is it even easier to lower the weight than to hold it and lift it? If you are producing the same output force in all three circumstances, why is there such a difference in effort?

Friction—The reason that you experience such a noticeable difference in required effort is in one instance of the exercise, friction is "hurting" you, in another instance there is *no friction* and in the last instance friction is "helping" you. But why is this so?

It is for the very same reason that, once a car starts to accelerate it does not speed off into infinity and why when you hit the brakes you are able to deaccelerate and eventually stop…in one instance friction prevents you from going faster than a certain speed, in the other it assists you in slowing down.

This in terms of exercise means that, when you are lifting a weight, friction is working against you and forcing your muscles to produce a much higher level of force to not only overcome the force of the weight but also friction. Therefore, while you maybe producing 100 pounds of "output" force—force that is capable of being used to perform productive work of some sort—your muscles are actually generating approximately 120 pounds of force—100 pounds to lift the weight plus 20 percent more to overcome friction. However, this friction only applies where there is motion, which means that if you were to merely hold that 100 pounds of resistance your muscles would be required to produce *exactly* 100 pounds…not an ounce more, not an ounce less. Although, if you were to begin to lower that weight, friction would rear its head again…only this time, you will be praising its name instead of cursing it. When you are lowering the weight, friction is acting in the same direction that your muscles are producing force. So while you are required to produce 100 pounds of output force, that same 20 percent of friction that hindered you while you were lifting the weight is actually adding to your strength while you are lowering it, so now while you are producing 100 pounds of output force your muscles are only required to generate 80 pounds of force.

However, this internal muscular friction is not undeviating…it changes. Two factors that change muscular friction are fatigue and repetition speed. The first is unavoidable, as you near momentary muscular failure, you accrue fatigue moment by moment and friction continues to build little by little in the muscles. But unless you fatigue your strength to the point where your positive strength is weakened so much that you are incapable of moving against less than one pound of resistance, the accruing friction as your muscles fatigue is negligible. On the other hand, speed of movement can increase muscular friction to a notable degree.

Increasing the speed of movement will increase muscular and joint friction, for the same reason that when you speedup your car you do not accelerate into infinity. The third law of motion states that to every action there is an equal and opposite reaction or in other words, everything that has mass and motion has friction (and since every entity of value in the universe has mass, even the smallest particle of dust to the planets and interstellar asteroids are delimited in there speed by friction).

When you accelerate a car, you will ultimately reach a maximal velocity when your car is incapable of producing any higher level of forward force. When you are producing a constant maximal force, the road and air will meet you head-on with an equal and opposite force, thus allowing you a terminal velocity of the car's maximum speed. Therefore, when you are attempting to make a lift easier towards the end of a set by moving faster (without compromising correct form) you are, in fact, only doing harm by increasing the amount of opposing force that you have to lift against, them's the facts. And although there are fools out there who will tell you that such an increase in force by accelerated lifting will expose your muscles to a greater force and thus overload the muscles being employed, using less weight and thus, according to them, being much safer, I will tell you here and now that such is utterly false, wrong, erroneous, foolish, stupid…pure insanity. And this is why….

Explosive Stupidity

Let's say that you contract your biceps, placing your upper arm in the fully contracted position, and then move your forearm by extending it, via the triceps, as fast as you can. Now you might be able to move your arm at 1500 to 2500 degrees per second—seeing that an individual's average range of motion for the elbow joint, from full extension to full contraction, is approximately 155 degrees. However, let's say you add resistance. You quickly realize that even with only using one pound of resistance you are incapable of moving your arm as fast as you did without resistance.

Furthermore, as you keep increasing the resistance you notice that the maximum speed you are able to produce drops significantly. Upon reaching the maximum weight you are able to contract against you will notice that the resulting speed created when trying to move the weight as fast as you are capable of is *zero*. You are only able to contract against it statically, possessing no power to accelerate the weight, that is, to move the resistance. Why? Because when you are moving as fast as you are capable, all of the force that your muscles are producing is directed solely at accelerating the mass of the limbs themselves. Add any resistance and you compromise the amount of force that you direct at the limb to move it faster.

When lifting in a positive manner with a meaningful weight you are *forced* to move slowly. You are moving the weight slowly because nearly every ounce of your muscular force capability is being used to move the resistance. Consequently, since most of your muscular strength is being used to move the weight you are usually incapable to accelerate up to a velocity that is faster than a 3 to 10 second pace.

When you are moving as fast as you can, you are, in fact, at your weakest. The faster you move the less lifting force you are capable of producing. When you are moving as fast as you are capable you are producing *zero* output force, as all of your power potential is being utilized to accelerate the limbs themselves, leaving nothing leftover to contract against any additional resistance.

In order to stimulate muscle growth you are required to *overload* the muscles with a meaningful resistance. If you are using a weight that is significant, only the first few repetitions will allow you to move at anything close to what you could call fast…but those are also the most dangerous repetitions. The last ones are by far the safest, since you are literally too weak to produce enough force to injure yourself. For this reason, the first few repetitions must be performed in a much slower manner than possible, since you are strongest at that time, but once you near the end of that set, trying to lift the weight as fast as you can becomes far safer since your ability to dramatically increase the force you can expose your connective tissues and joints to is significantly lower.

If your goal is to become a competitive weightlifter, you are required to perform the movements (the snatch and the clean & jerk) in such an explosive fashion. But doing so will do little for your strength…but the costs of such little gains are high. What you are doing is developing a skill, whether you know it or not, not muscular strength. To try to correlate such practices in bodybuilding exercise is utterly idiotic and just damn near insanity, as you will not be developing the muscular strength to lift a significant weight, but the *skill* to throw a significant weight via dangerous leveraging of the primary axes of the skeletal frame. Coinciding with the fact that you will be unsuccessfully overloading the muscles you are trying to target, as you are not lifting the weight with muscular power, since the joints and connective tissues are receiving most of the load. This is why you see so many older weightlifters—being as young as their 40's and 50's—are either in a wheel chair or semi-crippled with severe chronic back, knee and shoulder pain.

Knowing that, because Olympic-style weightlifters are a small and very defensive group of athletes (just like bodybuilders), there will no doubt be cries of outrage and protest against the previous statements. Nevertheless, those are the facts of the matter…and facts are just that: facts, neither my opinions nor speculations.

I have been a weightlifter when I was younger, my father is currently a weightlifter and trains with an accomplished champion weightlifter who holds a few records in his class….I have seen the injurious direct effects of explosive lifting firsthand…I am not talking about results at this time, which are not immediate but occur over a period of time, an effect is immediate, a direct resultant produced during or immediately after the situation. In my case, I got out of the activity before it completely ruined my shoulders… my father now has chronic, and sometimes, violent knee pain…the individual who my father trains with had a severe injury himself that nearly ended his career. I have witnessed weightlifting competitions via numerous videos, photos and firsthand. Despite what many strength and conditioning coaches or exercise physiology professors tell you at the universities and collages, the rate of injury for individuals who perform explosive lifting is very high. Don't get me wrong, I have a very high respect for a number of champion Olympic weightlifters; Paul Anderson, John Davis, Tommy Kono, John Grimek and Vasily Alexeev are all men that I have admired at one point or another, but the sport itself is just that, a sport, i.e. a *skill*, and until Olympic weightlifting comes to been seen for exactly what it is, instead of a method of attaining "explosive strength," there will be many more injuries to come, I promise you that.

* * *

If you are lifting truly heavy weights, which is mandatory if you desire to produce anything in the way of improvement, then you are forced to move slowly, it is literally impossible to move rapidly...you can throw it up pretty damn fast, but you are incapable of lifting it rapidly; and throwing weights will not do a damn thing for your strength.

I have seen individuals in the gym, for many years, use the entire stack on some machines, load up leg presses and grab the heavy dumbbells for curls, only to perform the exercises in such a stupid and dangerous fashion that crooked Chiropractors a couple of blocks away could feel their wallets start to grow.

...The results of their efforts you ask? Well if you are interested in their muscular results, many had upper arm and calf sizes that I could only compare to the size of my wrists. But if you are interested in their actual "gains," you would be better off asking their physicians...I cannot keep track of all the newly gained apparel consisting of knee, ankle and back braces that I've seen. The only thing that I can think of that comes close to such dangerous and injury assuring movements, besides running, would be plyometrics, which is a system of activity that is based on high impact force for resistance and lengthy repetitious activities...and if we lived in anything even approaching a relatively sane society, such individuals that perform plyometrics, ballistic weight lifting and marathon running for "health" benefits would be visited by the men in white, fitted into a snug long sleeved jacket and escorted to their local funny farm where they can be properly restrained from influencing the rest of society with their insanities...but the truth of the matter is that these are the individuals that are teaching the next generation what qualifies as "exercise"… what qualifies as "safe," as "productive."

What does this say about the state of the scientific community in the field of exercise? …The inmates are running the asylum.

And if a full understanding of everything up to this point leaves you feeling a little embarrassed for not having been previously aware of such obvious facts of reality, just know this. In the early 1900's, when the Wright brothers were performing almost daily flying demonstrations, there were still individuals in the scientific community that proclaimed that heavier than air flight was impossible… but apparently these individuals had never seen a bird before. Sure.

Don't be embarrassed by your mistakes…learn from them. Recall earlier I said that finding an individual that will admit a mistake, even if it is one that they have held for many years that resulted in countless hours wasted, will have you hard-pressed…but even more so when trying to find one that will actually learn from it…I hope that you who are reading this are one of those rare individuals.

Don't continue down a blind alley of tradition because of fear of being held accountable for your mistakes… if you have wasted thousands of dollars on expensive supplements and countless hours in the gym, stop! … Stop being a victim of volitional cowardice and cultural pressure to conform.

* * *

The first requisite of a proper productive exercise is high intensity and LOW FORCE…an exercise performed with a specific repetition cadence for the purpose of overloading the muscles with constant stress and no momentum. The speed of all of your repetitions ought to be conducted in a cadence with every single repetition performed in a deliberate fashion, that is, performed under full muscular control. In the positive or lifting phase of the movement you should be lifting at a speed that requires 4 to 5 seconds to reach the fully contracted position. Do not merely throw the weight up with improper form and accelerated lifting—lift it under control!

If there is a load on the muscle in the fully contracted position—examples are pulldowns, leg extensions, triceps cable extensions, calf raises, and dumbbell lateral raises—hold the weight statically for 2 seconds. If there is no load in the contracted position pause briefly and turnover before the skeletal frame is supporting the load for too long.

Finally, lower the weight in 4-5 seconds in the negative or lowering phase. *Do not drop the weight!* Studies have shown that the negative aspect of an exercise is the most beneficial for stimulating muscle growth. Once reaching the fully extended position do not pause there, smoothly begin the next repetition—again I repeat, never stop in the fully extended position. Just as momentum will allow recovery so too will resting in the fully extended position.

Following this cadence will eliminate any and all momentum—an outside force that will reduce the load on the muscle—and prevent force induced injuries that can vary from minor connective tissue damage to the complete rupture of connection tissues, requiring surgical attention. This cadence is vital if you are to successfully overload the muscles and avoid injury—specifically, you have to go slow!

The second requirement of a productive workout is

a smooth transition, of which, is a consequence of using no momentum. The necessity of this became evidently clear when I had one client perform a set of leg presses with a second-degree tear of his Calcaneofibular ligament induced two week prior. After a feeble attempt to detour him from significantly loading the injured ankle, I caved in…as he was quite insistent.

After sufficiently lowering the weight from his previous uses by approximately 35 percent, I repeated the severity of a slow repetition cadence and told him to tell me if he felt any "twinge" or slight discomfort—save for muscular discomfort of course. As he started the movement, I keep a close eye on his legs and one eye on his face in order to spot any facial grimacing telling of pain. When he was coming to the transition point, I noticed that he sped up in a quick reversing style and his facial musculature automatically cringed. Immediately I told him to end the set and slowly lower the weight. After questioning the severity of the pain in his ankle, I remembered an article written by Dr. Doug McGuff about this very situation and the importance of a smooth transition.

Upon recollection of this fact, I notified this individual that the pain was caused by a dramatic increase in force produced in his quick directional change in acceleration from the positive to the negative and that if he performed the movement in a smoother fashion there would be little to no pain. Thus, after asking if he was comfortable with attempting another set, he again set himself in the proper position and smoothly initiated the set. As he was coming to the transition I kept a close eye on his face again; smoothly he transitioned into the negative portion of the movement and exclaimed upon questioning, "Didn't feel a thing."

Wraps and Suits and Shirts! Oh, My!

When I was first introduced to the iron game at the age of ten, I entered into a world of heavy stiff leg deadlifting, brutal bench presses and excruciating military presses. However, even though I was deeply invested in the works of strength, it was not until much later that I knew that many lifters use lifting straps, knee and elbow wraps, lifting belts and lifting shirts and suits. My longtime impression was that these tools were used for preventing injury and/or protecting an individual who was already injured...boy was I wrong.

There are many weightlifters, powerlifters and strongmen who utilize these tools for their intended purpose...but there are countless bodybuilders who use them when they are damn near worthless to the bodybuilder. The primary goal of the competent bodybuilder is to become progressively stronger...*not* to demonstrate their strength.

Though it may be difficult for many to distinguish the difference between "training for strength" and "demonstrating strength," there is an important distinction. Demonstrating strength, as seen in powerlifting, strongman and Olympic weightlifting competitions, is the act of lifting the most weight you can one to three times... getting the weight up in any manner required. Training for strength is performing an exercise in the proper manner, without sacrificing form, to the point where you are unable to perform another repetition and then attempting to perform more repetitions, utilize more weight or both the next workout...utilizing a sub-maximal weight to weaken the targeted muscles.

What wraps, suits and shirts allow you to do is to

"lift" more weight *in spite* of your strength....Have you ever notice that when you compress a spring, and then all of a sudden release it, that it violently extends back to its original state or when you release the trigger of a catapult, it hurls objects an appreciable distance. What we are dealing with in these situations is the very same thing that is found when you see someone wrap up their knees and elbows or put on a lifting suit or shirt before a lift...there is potential or stored energy. Stored energy is "potential" work or force. When you compress a spring, you are putting kinetic energy into the spring—kinetic energy is the energy that was needed to accelerate an object to a certain velocity. When you have compressed the spring as far as possible, you have put in a certain potential of energy that is stored until the spring is unopposed by an object that has an inertia that is greater than its potential force...and since air friction is relatively low, the spring with violently return to its original position once you remove your hand.

When an individual wraps up his knees or elbows for a lift, he is essential wrapping a spring around his joints. During the negative aspect of the lift, the chosen weight that is being used stores energy in the material of the knee and elbow wraps...but a nonresistant material does not store energy—when you compress a spring it becomes progressively harder as even the smallest unit of stored energy that is put in at the start is attempting to escape in the opposite direction that you are applying force, with every little bit more put in opposing your efforts. Because of the material's tendency to oppose the force that is putting energy into it, in this case the weight of the barbell or machine, the resistance on the muscles is less than it would be without the wraps…in some cases it can be significantly less.

Now when he begins his ascent to his original position, the stored energy has only one way to go… and that means that the wraps actually help him lift the weight, requiring less muscular effort than would otherwise be required. The lifting suits and shirts do the same…make you look strong, but do not a damn thing for your strength. The purpose of strength training is exposing your muscles to progressively heavier loads… wraps allow you to lift more weight, but only expose your bones, tendons and ligaments to useless, potentially dangerous, excessive weights.

Unless used in serious lifting competitions for the purpose of moving the most weight possible, these tools only feed the insecurities of what I used to call "the little big man syndrome." What I refer to when I say the little big man syndrome is a larger than average male who has an inferiority complex to every other person in the gym with a scrotum and feels the absolute need to move more weight than anyone so he can preserve his "masculinity" among the very few real and many imaginary people who actually give a damn about what he does in the gym… essential an imitation of an animal pissing all over the place to mark his "territory."

My advice for anyone who wants to obtain the most from their efforts in the gym, even though you won't initially be lifting as much weight as you could if you sacrificed form and use lifting ads, is to ignore everyone else in the gym, leave the wraps, lifting shirts and suits at home, do not sacrifice form for weight and smarten up.

Keep Breathing and Stay Still Damn it!

As aggressive a title as any I suppose…but one that adequately allows the reader to grasp how severely I take the subject at hand. The third requirement is that the individual training breathes properly throughout the exercise.

Most individuals when performing a high intensity muscular exertion will hold their breath and perform the Val Salva maneuver—this is neither recommended nor desired, as the Val Salva maneuver can be extremely dangerous. Many bodybuilders, powerlifters and weightlifters perform the Val Salva maneuver, and a notable number have had an aneurysm burst…and when you are balancing 300 to 600 pounds over your chest, it is not exactly the most convenient time for such to happen. Upon initiation of the set, breathing should be calm and controlled; as the intensity begins to rise the speed of your breathing should follow suit; when in the last and most intense phase of the set breathing should be calm but rapid…essentially the main concern to keep the airway open.

The fourth requirement of a productive workout is control and sedation of the extremities and facial musculature. During a high intensity workout, most individuals have the tendency of flailing their extremities, grimacing and yelling for emotional comfort, physical detraction from the muscular discomfort or just in an attempt to convey that they are training harder than they actually are. These activities are neither desirable nor productive, as gripping hard when not required raises blood pressure to an undesirable level. (Your circulatory system is a closed hydraulic system. If you close off any part of it by clenching your teeth or by squeezing the handles of a machine your blood pressure skyrockets and it could result in medical problems, such as blowing of an aneurysm.)

The biggest reason for avoidance of these activities is exemplified by looking at a *Cortical Homunculus*. A Cortical Homunculus is a physical representation of the primary motor cortex of the brain that is responsible for physical movement. Now certain quantities of the brain's motor cortex is devoted to a certain body part and the larger the area of brain that is devoted to that aspect of the body the more neurological activity is used in its functioning. For example, let us say that you are performing a heavy set of leg presses and you grip the handles greatly, yell and make a face that is only warranted by breaking your leg. Your thighs and hips require only a tiny percentage of the brains neurological activity, but your hands, face and the musculature used for vocalization use approximately 80 percent of the motor cortex in order to function. The massive neural discharge from this section of the brain comes down and can potentially wash over the signal you are trying to send to your hips and thighs and may result in you suddenly failing.

Although it is difficult not to do these things, just attempt to avoid these activities…a moan or a slight grimace occasionally won't hurt you if you can't help it. But there is a lot to be said about a man training at super high intensities, with hundreds of pounds, expressing only the stoic face of an intense focus. As my father once said to me, "It is the quiet ones who come out of nowhere and blow everyone away without making any noise, with no expression, that are the ones that people start to talk about with awe and reverence."

The Training Journal

The fifth requirement of a productive training program is a training journal. The training journal is your key to knowing that your training efforts are not in vain. How do you know if you are training properly if you do not record your workouts? Most muscle enthusiast will go straight for the scale before a workout to see if they have gained any muscle. If they have not gained weight these individuals become unsettled and stand there wondering, "Why am I not gaining any muscle?" The problem is that muscle growth on a day-to-day basis or even weekly is agonizingly slow for most individuals... more often than not, most will have no gain in muscular size over a period of time and then, literally almost over night, they will gain a few pounds or more of muscle. So tracking your progress by taking daily body measurements and weighing yourself everyday is utterly useless. Even if you used the most advanced tools available today for composition measurements and changes in bodily girth measurements, they can be extremely misleading as many individuals gain muscle mass cyclically, growing continually stronger for a period of time and then an increase in mass to facilitate greater strength.

Others will insist that it is the pump or how sore you are after a workout that indicates whether you have stimulated growth or not. This, however, is as erroneous a notion as any, as neither the pump nor soreness is indicative of growth stimulation. Jump down on your stomach pump out 30 rapid-fire push-ups, stand up, look in the mirror and you will find that you have an appreciable pump in your chest and arms...but did you stimulate any muscle growth? Of course not.

If the pump were indicative of muscle growth than hundreds of thousands of bewildered bodybuilders, all around the world, would be in possession of 20 inch arms, a 60 inch chest and 30 inch legs. As for muscle soreness, the term muscle soreness is actually an oxymoron. The contractile tissues of the muscle do not possess the type of nerves required to indicate pain. What is actually transmitting the feeling of a dull pain (or soreness) is actually what is called C-fibers, which are located primarily in the connective tissues where the muscle and tendon join. Furthermore, many individuals have actually gone months, working out intensely and infrequently, but have not had any muscular soreness during that time...but they progressed nonetheless.

In order to make sure that you are training in a continuously productive manner, you require a standard that is accurate and is universally applicable. And since we have already established that muscular size is interrelated to muscular strength, we know that for a program to be productive you must be getting stronger every workout, in either reps, weight or both—your standard is your strength gains.

The point I am trying to make is that you must keep a training journal for the same reason as a doctor keeps a medical chart of his patients. A doctor can better advise you with a medical chart, recording your past medical history, to the same degree that you too can better direct your training efforts by making the necessary adjustments to accommodate signs of a slow in progress and your dynamic recovery needs.

* * *

The only way you will know if you are training correctly is if you are getting stronger. It is impossible to evaluate something without measurement. There is no guesswork in engineering, astronautics or surgery and neither should there be in your training.

Before each workout, you need to record the exercises that you will be performing, the date and, if desired, your bodyweight—this comes in handy more when an individual is on a weight loss program. The weight and repetitions performed on each exercise must be recorded as well.

Training Beyond Positive Failure... A Double-edged Sword?

The predicament of the high intensity training methodology at this point in time is that most hardcore "HIT" enthusiasts feel the utter need to train as hard as possible and are always trying to produce a greater degree of muscular stimulation. As a result, in their pursuit of more muscle mass, they perform advance high intensity protocols that deepen the inroading of the exercises... sometimes to tremendous degrees. However, the problem with this approach is that it accumulates the equivalent result as high volume training, in which you overwhelm the body's recovery ability and overdose on the stimulus. And just as with any kind of stimulus you have, as described by Dr. Doug McGuff with his dose-response relationship to exercise, a therapeutic window. With higher intensities of the stimulant you create a narrower and narrower therapeutic window of gaining positive results and a greater chance of toxicity and of causing harm.

Though the recommendation of the distorted HIT community is to perform exercise to a degree of the highest possible intensity, I have learned, through much trial and error, that such practices with higher intensity protocols (i.e. rest-pause, negative-only, negative accentuated and even something as low-grade as forced reps) will do little in the way of improving the average individual's strength training program, for an advanced bodybuilder or athlete, sure...but for the average walking past you on the street, it has the eventual potential of doing a lot more harm to their results than good. Though the up held wisdoms of the HIT community held that there was the requirement of higher intensity protocols for the more advanced bodybuilder, such an action of switching from a stick of dynamite to an atomic bomb *will* greatly increase the destructive potential of your efforts (an excellent analogy when you take into consideration that exercise is a negative factor on the body)....But, when the goal is to clear a path through a mountain and not to completely eradicate the damn thing of the face of the planet, you come to see the non-necessity of increasing the potency of your tool. Remember that the aim is precision in inroading the muscle, not to kill yourself in your efforts. Positive failure, i.e. taken to the point where you are literally incapable of producing even the slightest fraction of an inch of progressive movement, is all that is usually necessary. Even a few forced reps have the potential of increasing the inroad of that muscle from a productive 20 or so percent to a degree that crosses over the threshold of productiveness into detriment.

There does exist a threshold within all of our physiologies that holds a distinct temperament, one that dictates how much intensity/volume is profitable and at what point it becomes overkill. And although this threshold varies in degree between individuals, it cannot be ignored…not if you want to train in a productive manner. In studying the benefit of regular and irregular use of advanced high intensity protocols, I have formed the opinion that not only are advanced techniques like infitonic training, Omni contraction training and negative accentuated not profitable for about 90 percent of trainees, but that they are, more often than not, counterproductive.

The proper approach to an intelligent and productive training program is only performing exactly, or as close to as possible, the correct amount of exercise required, equally in terms of volume, frequency and *intensity*, for the purpose of eliciting a response with the least amount of physiologic resources exhausted. In using advance high intensity protocols such as rest-pause and negative-only, once you have been training with regular high intensity, positive failure exercise for a year or more, if you are seeing that you are treading your potential, you can use them sporadically if you choose to do so…but NEVER in the barbell squat nor in the deadlift. You can play with fire all you want…but doing so with exercises that have a potential inherit risk factor of kerosene WILL increase the very low risk of potential of properly performed squats and deadlifts to a very high one…the spine can only take so much compressive force. However, do not be afraid to add an additional rest day or more in order to compensate from their greater physiologic demand.

It is up to you to monitor and regulate your training. Most, if not all, individuals reading this possess the requisite intelligence needed for achieving their physical potential…but it is up to you to apply your reason to the realm of your goals and desires.

Confidence and Patience

We come to the final requisite in your training that is, in my firm opinion, the single most important factor in your production of the best possible gains in muscular size and strength. Confidence and patience are usually intertwine: in order to be patient you must be confident that you are not just wasting your time…in being confident you know that what you desire is possible and you are doing everything possible to obtain it, so you are patient.

It is my opinion that the single most downfall of anyone who starts on a bodybuilding routine is a lack of confidence…but this is not always a bad thing, it means that you are unsure of the information that you are being dealt and do not hold it with full conviction. If you were one of the many individuals who experience a lack of confidence when attempting one of the routines espoused in the magazines, I would say that this more of a blessing over a flaw. Of course trying a routine that is backed up by equivocations and fallacy is difficult to trust. However, even when introduced to a rational approach to bodybuilding exercise, several individuals still frantically run about, impatient.

Why is this? It is because they do not fundamentally grasp the theory and lack a keystone that causes them to become impatient…soon to lack confidence.

How do I know? I was one of them. I fully grasped the theory myself, applied it to the training efforts of my clients and training partners…I completely grasped the theoretical, but I mistakenly, unknowingly, moronically, detached it from my own practical efforts in the gym… like I said before, I have not been the smartest person in the world at times.

In the next chapter I will make mention of the few of the grave mistakes that I have made that might help you avoid repeating my mistakes, but one that is imperative and is the single most cause for this widespread plague of impatience and lack of confidence must be addressed at this time.

Since our main concern as bodybuilders is to build the greatest amount of muscle mass possible, bodybuilders, in general, have accumulated a rather large amount of emotional investment towards acquiring muscle in the fastest manner possible. Therefore, when a bodybuilder is investing his time and efforts in a method of exercise and is getting none of that "now" muscle…he usually becomes anxious. The problem in this case is that he is assessing his progress by secondary means. Remember that muscle growth is a secondary…it is caused by a need to grow stronger than the currently available cross-sectional area of muscle. Muscle growth, as was explained earlier, is a very inaccurate way to assess one's progress.

As I have mentioned before, and I will mention again later on, there is an interdependent relationship between muscular size and strength. As long as you are becoming stronger, you will eventually grow larger. If you start out deadlifting 150 pounds for ten reps and then after a few months of training are able to deadlift 300 pounds for fifteen reps, although we cannot calculate precisely how much stronger you have become, there has unquestionably been a change in your physiology that has allowed for this much greater strength.

Worrying about muscle growth when your concern should be gradual, consistent, strength increases will only cause you the harm of increased stress levels and divest you of the confidence that you are going to gain size if you train hard...thus you lose the confidence that your values are not unreachable, in addition to losing certainty of your efforts, resulting in half-assed efforts in the gym since most do not want to discomfort themselves with hard work when they don't know if it is worth the effort.

Concern yourself with becoming stronger—the size will come.

8

Concretization of the Theory

The purpose of the previous chapters was to acquire the *theoretical knowledge* required to guide you successfully in *practical* action. This chapter will be dealing with a concretization of the theory of high intensity training in accord with the theoretical foundation that you have acquired. Thus, this chapter is going to depict the *ideal bodybuilding routine* for nearly everyone, no matter their genetically predisposed muscular mass potential or their distinctive recovery needs.

An ideal bodybuilding routine is one that is designed to be consonant with all of the fundamental principles that permit the stimulation and growth of optimal muscular development. The routines must be of high intensity—this, of course, lies solely on the trainee's effort. Secondly, the routine must be of a low enough volume as to not overwhelm the recovery faculties of the body's growth mechanism. Thirdly, the routine must be of a low enough frequency to allow time required to both recover from the exhaustive effects of the workout and to fully overcompensate, once fully recovered, with muscle growth.

In order to allow the second need we must choose only the exercises that are the most productive for complete systemic stimulation. The following exercises are the most beneficial exercises that are available in virtually every gym or fitness center and these selected exercises will facilitate total systemic stimulation of all major muscle groups.

The Squat

If you want big legs, you will have to start to love the squat. No other exercise will stimulate the degree of growth in the thighs and hips that the squat is capable of. The squat is one of the two most productive and systemically stimulating exercises that an individual can perform. I am not overstating this even slightly when I say that, the squat and the deadlift will stimulate muscular growth that is unparallel to any other form or combination of exercises. The squat requires an enormous amount of exertion from the gluteus, the quadriceps, the hamstrings, and the musculature of the core. This exercise can be performed with either with a smith machine or a barbell in a power rack.

The performance of the squat is fairly simple: first, you must approach the bar and set yourself under. The bar should rest across your shoulders and set below the nape of your neck—if a pad is needed make sure it is not so thick that it applies pressure on your neck. Set your feet shoulder width apart, feet pointing slightly outwards. Begin descending from a standing position keeping your head up throughout the entire exercise, chin parallel to the floor or higher and keep your back straight or even concave. Start by pushing your hips slightly behind you and then begin bending your knees. Descend to the point where there your hamstrings are touching your calf muscles or as close to as possible. *Do not drop into the rock bottom position* with your buttocks flush against you calves and then bounce back up. Doing so will only guarantee injury; remember this is high intensity, *low force* exercise. Once reaching the point where your hamstrings are touching your calves, without ever stopping in the bottom position, begin to slowly, under full muscular control, ascending back to the starting position. When rising back to the top position, blow out the air in your lungs and lift your chest and head up—this will help prevent you from leaning too far forward. Pause briefly in the top position, pausing only long enough to take in a deep breath, and then begin the next repetition.

There is no need to perform half squats with the false perception that they are "safer"…they are not. The full barbell squat, performed deliberately and without any explosive lifting or bouncing, is far more beneficial than a half squat, a partial squat or any other type you wish to confer. The full squat is more beneficial since it reduces the amount of weight that you can handle because you are moving through a much greater range of motion… why is this better? When you use the super heavy weights that are possible in partial squats, due to the superior leverage advantage of the bones, you are exposing your lumbar spine to an immense degree of stress. And while the full squat makes it very difficult to use super heavy weight, you are actually exposing your quadriceps and buttocks to a much greater intensity and *resistance* than would otherwise be exposed to your muscles with the half or partial squat.

…A Paradox? Not by any means…it is simple physics. Remember that gravity is fixed and constant…it acts in only direction (which is down) and pulls everything on earth with a constant force. When you are lifting a barbell, gravity is acting on that barbell constantly and in only one direction, straight down, but you are lifting through one or more rotations.

When performing a barbell squat, since we are dealing with movement around an axis, in this case the knee, hip and ankle, we are dealing with torque. Torque is established by multiplying the moment arm or lever (which is the distance from the point where the force is acting upon the lever to the axis) by the force acting upon the moment arm (torque equals lever arm times force). In the start of the squat, we will make this barbell weigh exactly 100 pounds, the horizontal distance of the moment arm is zero, and therefore the force acting upon the hips and thighs is zero. If you were to have your knees locked in the fully contracted position, you could literally hold up the universe, if your bones, ligaments and tendons were strong enough…and your muscles would not even be aware of it, because even an infinity amount of resistance times zero is still zero. As you descend with the barbell, after 30 degrees of movement the moment arm has increased (the latitudinal distance from the knees to the hips) and there is now force acting upon the quadriceps and buttocks…but while gravity is acting in a downward direction, because force that is acting upon the thighs is acting in a different, rotational, direction, and you are not a position where gravity is able to act on your muscles directly, you are only exposing your thighs to only part of that one hundred pounds.

Once you reach the point where your thighs are parallel to the floor, knees bent at approximately 110 to 120 degrees, you are at the only position where your muscles are forced to contract against 100 pounds...your thighs are forced to act against gravity in exactly the opposite direction of its pull and you are in the position where the moment arm is at its greatest length. After you pass that position, the resistance exposed to your thighs begins to decease again until you reach full flexion of the knee where the moment arm is shorter and approximately 45 degrees away from a perpendicular position...depending on one's respective body leverage factors.

If you were to perform only partial repetitions or half squats (where the knee is bent just short of 90 degrees), using a significant enough weight to get the attention of your muscles, you are exposing your bones, ligaments and tendons to the much greater force that an advantageous leverage allows...but you have done little to expose your muscles to a greater resistance that could have be more effectively and safely gained through full range squats. Reaching the point where your thighs are parallel to the floor and lower, you are moving through the most beneficial and productive area of the squat. The top five inches of the squat are useless in terms of stimulating muscle growth...your muscles are barely aware of anything, but if you are using in excess of 500 or 700 pounds, you can be damn sure that your lumbar, thoracic and cervical spine, your knees and your hips are aware of something.

Most people steer clear of full squats because they believe that full squats are dangerous for the knees. Well sure, I suppose that putting 300 pounds on your back and relaxing your hips and thighs as you unlock your knees would do something decidedly unpleasant...but I bet that doing the same while walking down a flight of stairs will not be any more productive for your knees. Of course full squats can be dangerous…driving your car can be dangerous, picking up a child can be dangerous, hell, even brushing your damn teeth can be dangerous…but the danger is almost always in someone doing something decidedly stupid. Dropping into the rock bottom position during heavy full squats *will* hurt your knees—there is no maybe in this situation, this is a guarantee—whether you are able to walk away after or do not suffer from knee pain currently is irrelevant, you will do some degree of damage to your knees.

If you perform the full squat in the fashion described above you will not injure your knees…you will however be doing a hell of a lot in the way of preventing future knee injury by strengthening the musculature around the knee. The real reason that most avoid the full squat is twofold. Firstly, doing full squats, especially if you have not been doing them before, does not allow for the same poundage as the partial squat…hurting their little big man syndrome. Secondly, and what is the main causal deterrent, if you do them right, they are probably one of the hardest things you will ever do in life…they are harder than nearly every other exercise, save for the deadlift. Due to their difficulty—not in spite of it, but a direct result of their difficulty—they will stimulate levels of muscular size nearly unattainable by any other exercise or combination of exercises. If you want bigger arms and pecs (the most favored of body parts among neophytes), you are going to have to train legs. Upper body growth will be limited if you don't.

The incredible benefits that squats are capable of

bestowing are yours to reap, but the momentary costs are high…however it's ultimately up to you whether you bite the bullet and endure the brief duration of insistent ache or you can wimp out and give up on your goals because of momentary discomfort.

A cruel statement…sure…but as I said to one individual when he read a few lines in my book and retorted that I was coming off a bit callous, "What bodybuilders need nowadays is not another fool posing as their 'buddy,' but cold hard facts…the truth."

<u>Palms-Up Pulldowns</u>

The palms-up pulldown (or chin-up) is one of the— if not the—most productive upper body exercises. It requires the exertion of the forearm flexors, the biceps, the triceps, the deltoids, the latissimus dorsi, the trapezius, the rhomboids, the teres major, the pectorals, and the abdominals. The underhand pulldown, besides being the greatest latissimus exercise, is in fact the greatest biceps exercise there is, without a doubt.

In order to perform the pulldown place your hands slightly within your shoulder width. Have your palms fully supinated facing towards yourself in an underhand or what is known as a curling grip fashion. This is very important as the biceps will only be fully stimulated when the palms are completely supinated. When the palms are moved into a pronated position the much smaller and weaker brachialis is used as the main flexor of the elbow. This hinders the maximum strength of the arm and mitigates the latissimus and the biceps from receiving sufficient stimulation.

Now with your palms supinated and placed slightly

within shoulder width, sit down with your knees sliding underneath the thigh pads or have a seat belt fully secure. Then with a smooth initiation, pull the bar down into the fully contracted position at your clavicle. Once reaching the position of full contraction were the bar is at the same height as your clavicle pause for two long seconds and then slowly begin returning to the position of *full* extension. Then without pausing, without jerking, smoothly begin your next repetition.

<u>Dips</u>

Coined as the upper body squat, dips are the greatest exercise for stimulating the pectorals and the triceps... just look at Olympic Gymnasts like Yang Wei who possesses shoulders and arms that are more impressive than many top-ranked bodybuilders' are. He developed those impressive shoulders and arms with his work on the parallel bars. However, dips are not only the greatest triceps and pectoral exercise there is but also an extremely productive shoulder exercise as well. The dip fulfills all functions of the pectorals and the triceps and, as it works through the shoulder axis, the deltoids contribute greatly in this exercise.

Many trainees stray away from dips in favor of the long time favorite, the bench press. But, although the barbell bench press can be a very productive exercise if utilized correctly, it does not approach the prodigious capabilities of the dip.

To begin, take hold of the handles on a set of dipping bars and press yourself up to the lockout position so that your arms support your body weight. Slowly lower yourself down until you feel a comfortable stretch in your pectoral muscles and then, without pausing, slowly press yourself to the starting position. Have your uppers arms flare out away from the torso a bit.

Most modern gyms have specialized dipping machines with a selectorized weight stack to one side— where you sit on a seat and press down in a dipping fashion. This is great for those who are not yet strong enough to dip their own body weight or have shoulder pain while performing regular parallel bar dips (I highly recommend the Hammer Strength, MedX or Nautilus versions of the dip machine, if you have access to these models, take advantage of them). If you do not have access to such machines, and are momentarily too weak to perform regular dips, perform the negative-only method prescribed in the description of chin-ups.

On this exercise as well as the chin-up, you will quickly discover that your bodyweight becomes inadequate to support your muscle's increasing needs. Most gyms have what is called a dipping belt that can allow you to strap on more weight to further your training intensity or if you are training at a home gym or if you gym does not have one you can purchase one off a variety of online stores for a relatively inexpensive cost.

Standing Calf Raises

The proper technique to develop the calves is to perform a standing calf raise with the knees lock and the legs straight. This is a requirement of the gastrocnemius as this muscle originates from above the knee and it can only be fully contracted in a position in which the knee is fully locked and the ankle fully flexed. To demonstrate this, sit down on a chair with your knees bent and have your index finger placed on the muscle belly of the gastrocnemious—notice as you raise your heel up that the gastrocnemious does not contract.

The standing calf raise is very simple exercise. You can perform it on a leg press, as long as you keep you knees locked, or on a standing calf raise machine. But if neither are available, perform one-legged calf raises while holding a dumbbell in the hand that is on the same side as the calf that is doing the work, with your free arm grasping something sturdy for balance—the one legged calf raise is a very productive exercise that is much underrated.

From a position of full extension—your maximal range of descent—begin slowly ascending to the position of full contraction. This position is achieved best by visualizing yourself trying to reach the tip of your big toe, as a ballerina would do…after performing four or five repetitions in good form, when you reach as high as you think you can go, try hitching up another one or two inches. Then after reaching the position of full contraction pause for two to four seconds and then slowly begin descending back to the position of full extension, then, without pausing, initiate the next repetition.

Military Press

The military press works all three deltoid heads, the trapezius, and the triceps. There are many shoulder pressing machines, the greatest options being the pressing component of the Nautilus double shoulder machine, MedX shoulder press and the Hammer Strength Iso-lateral shoulder press.

If your only options are a smith machine or a barbell, take a shoulder-width grip and keep the elbows flared out so that the resistance is directly onto the deltoids as much as possible. From a position just above your clavicle, perform the movement slowly by pushing the bar over your head, pausing at the lockout just for a brief moment before lowering under control. After reaching the bottom position, begin the next repetition without bouncing or pausing.

The Deadlift

The Deadlift *is* the most productive exercise that you can perform for total systemic muscular stimulation. It does however possess some risk factors not seen elsewhere. Caution must be exercised when performing the barbell Deadlift—as with all exercises, but in particular the squat and the deadlift. The Deadlift requires the exertion of almost all of the muscles of the posterior aspect of the body, from the gastrocnemius of the calf to the trapezius of the neck. This exercise, along with the full squat, will, if performed properly, produce degrees of muscular development that are unprecedented when compared to any other exercise that exists, or may ever exist…but it is also one of the most physically and psychologically demanding. But man is it ever worth it when the deadlift can built such astonishing back development as that of Bob Peoples and Mark Berry.

To begin, position yourself in front of the bar with at least one 45 pound plate on each side, as to prevent you from over-stressing your lower back. Set your feet shoulder width apart. Then place your hands slightly outside the width of your shoulders with your hands placed in an interlocking grip with your dominate hand under or in what is known as a curling grip and your other hand placed over with your palm facing towards yourself.

Now, with the bar flush against your shins, bend at the hips and the knees to reach the bar and—this is critically important—*keep your back straight*, even concaved, having your shoulders *always* higher than your hips and your head up, the entire time. With your arms perfectly straight, with no jerking or pulling, slowly lift the bar with the mindset of trying to push your feet through the floor in order to stand up. Now once reaching the position of full contraction, without arching backwards, pause briefly, then slowly reverse the lift, and return to the bar to the floor. Once the bar is in the starting positions regrip the bar if necessary, take a deep breath and perform the next repetition.

Substitution Exercises

<u>Leg Press</u>

This exercise can be substituted for the squat if needed, as the leg press relieves the stress on the lower back and can be used as a substitute if your bodily leverages are not favorable for squats. The leg press is a very simple exercise that is performed in a range very similar to the squat, however when descending down into the position of full extension be careful not to raise your lower back off from the pad. Though the leg press lacks the degree of the squat's productiveness, it does possess the potential of stimulating growth to a degree that is still staggering when compared to almost any other form of exercise.

Begin by placing your feet approximately shoulder width on the foot plate of the machine and, if you are not using a MedX, Hammer strength or Nautilus leg press and are using a 45 degree or vertical leg press instead, place your hands on your knees. Do not perform repetitions using both your arms and your legs. Your hands are on your knees only allow you to return the sled to the top after your hips and thighs reach failure, you can use the additional strength of your arms to prevent the weight from descending down with your knees behind your ears. Use your hands after failure to push the weight back up to rack it once you reach failure.

Rows

The row is the favorite type of exercise for the musculature of the back among most bodybuilders. One made famous by an illustrious Mr. Olympia is what is called the Yates row...an exercise that many accredit to Dorian Yates' tremendous back muscularity. Now, although I very much doubt that his extraordinary back development was due to that exercise, it does not diminish the fact that the row can develop one's back significantly.

The row can be an extremely productive exercise that can be used as a substitute for or alternated with the pulldown or chins. It can be performed with a barbell, a dumbbell, a low cable pulley or a specially designed machine. If you have access to a Nautilus low friction row, a MedX row, a Pendulum 3-way row or a Hammer Strength iso-lateral "mid" row, utilize one of these machines over any manner of cable, barbell or dumbbell row. These machines are excellent and allow you to train your back far more efficiently than otherwise...just make sure not to lift your chest off the pad and remember to pull your elbows as far behind you and really squeeze your shoulder blades together for two seconds before lowering.

If your only options are a barbell or dumbbell, you can still get a terrific back workout if you perform the exercise properly. With a barbell, take an overhand grip that is slightly wider than shoulder width and bend at the hips, keeping your back flat the entire time. Keep your knees bent during the exercise to relieve tension on your lumbar spine. With your arms straight and both back and head parallel to the floor, pull the bar up until you touch your lower chest. Due to the mechanics of this exercise, it is exceedingly difficult to hold the fully contracted position, therefore, once reaching the top position, do not pause, but continue to lower the weight under control.

If you have access to dumbbells and a barbell, use a dumbbell instead of a barbell...it is far more efficient. With the dumbbell, bend over at the hips with one arm on a bench and grasp a dumbbell with the other. Now from full extension, pull the dumbbell up to your nipple area and, since you have the ability for a greater range of motion, make sure that your elbow passes the plane of your body, then hold for two seconds before lowering slowly. Perform as many repetitions as possible until failure and then switch sides.

Bench Press

This is the most popular and well-known exercise there is. This exercise can be used as a substitute for the dip if you lack the upper body strength for proper form or if your gym lacks a dip machine or a weight belt that allows you to utilize more weight in order to increase intensity. However, if you are able to do dips I recommend you do them, as they are a far more productive exercise than the bench press.

The bench press can be performed with a specialized machine, a barbell or on a smith machine. It is performed by lying flat on a bench and grasping the bar with a shoulder width grip, having your elbows flared out in order to allow for a full range of motion of the pectorals. (Contrary to what most bodybuilders believe, the pectorals do not obtain a greater stretch with a wide grip—just like in the pulldown—and in using a wide grip they are actually prevented from fulfilling the pectorals' main function. The major function of the pectorals is to draw the upper arm across the midline of the torso. To see the inefficiency with a wide grip, pretend you are doing a wide grip bench press. When you fully straighten your arm how close is your upper arm to the midline of your body? Now move your hands to your shoulder width. With your elbows flared out move your hands from full extension to contraction. Notice how great of a stretch there is in your pectorals in the fully extended position and how close your pectorals come to completing their main function in full contraction when you use a shoulder width grip.)

To begin the exercise, grasp the bar or handles with your thumbs around the bar—this must be done for all exercises in order prevent your hands from slipping and dissuade possibly injury. Unrack the bar and slowly lower the bar or handles down to your mid to lower chest and then once at your chest, without pausing, slowly begin ascending back to the position of full contraction, pausing briefly before beginning the next repetition.

Chin-ups

Chip-ups are performed in the same manner as pulldown, however, if you are initially too weak to perform chin-ups with your own bodyweight, start with negative-only chins. To perform negative-only chins place a bench or a chair next to the chin-up bar that is high enough so you can step off the chair into the top position where your chip is above the bar. Step up onto the chair, dismount into the top position, and hold that position for two seconds, then start to lower yourself very slowly, taking five to ten seconds to reach the fully extended position. If you are only able to perform one negative-only repetition at first do not become disheartened, with negative repetitions you will find that your strength increases will be dramatic and rapid.

Upon reaching the bottom position, reassume the top position as fast as possible and perform another repetition until you are unable to control your downward descent. Once you are capable of performing seven or more negative-only repetitions in a very slow manner you should be capable of performing full range positive repetitions.

The Program

Routine #1

Workout A
1. Squat—12-20 (alternate periodically with Leg Press)
2. Dips—6-10
3. Palms-up Pulldown—6-10

Workout B
1. Deadlift—8-15
2. Military Press—6-10
3. Standing Calf Raise—12-20

Repeat the cycle after workout B.

Routine #2 (Mike Mentzer's definitive Consolidated Routine)
Workout A
1. Squat—12-20 (alternate periodically with Leg Press)
2. Palms-up Pulldown—6-10

Workout B
1. Deadlift—8-15
2. Dips—6-10

Repeat the cycle after workout B.

Important Points

1. *Number of Sets:* Keep in mind that bodybuilding exercise science is a derivative of medical science, thus, possessing the same central requisite for precision. The point is not to do more or less—if more is 100 sets, which amounts to tremendous, gross overtraining, and doing less is doing half by performing 50 sets, which still amounts to severe overtraining, then you are still performing an arbitrary program based on just doing less then them or more then others. The issue is about performing the precise amount of exercise required to stimulate muscle growth, no more, no less. Let me restate that, since it is so vitally important in your efforts of productive bodybuilding exercise, *it is about performing the precise amount of exercise required to stimulate muscle growth, no more, no less.*

Now since the science of bodybuilding exercise is literally about achieving a high intensity muscular contraction we only concern ourselves with the only part of the exercise, the only repetition that requires a 100 percent high intensity muscular contraction: the last one. With that one last repetition completed, or just barely missed, you effectively turn on the growth mechanism of the body. Any more sets and you compromise that last repetition's potential, any less sets and there is no stimulus for muscle growth. Therefore, for each of the exercises listed perform one set of high intensity exercise to the point of momentary muscular failure.

2. *Volume & Frequency:* Over years of deliberation and study, Mike Mentzer found that a training frequency of once every 5-7 days was almost a miracle in the progress of almost all of his clients. Through the Haircut

study and in many other cases in my research I have come to appreciate and respect the body's physiologic adaptation mechanism. And if you seek to achieve your full muscular potential, you too must come to respect its nature's requirements. If you were to stroll over to your local grocery store, go into the meat section and pickup a pound of beef steak you would see that if you are asking your body to produce that, in addition to supporting all of the muscle you already have and performing all of its other countless metabolic processes, you are going to have to give it time to do so.

So when commencing your bodybuilding program, begin with routine one and begin with a training frequency of once every five to seven days. If you come to a point where you are not increasing the weight and/or reps for two cycles, take one to two weeks off and resume your training with one or two extra rest days inserted between workouts. Now from this point, when you observe—while consulting your training journal—that your progress is starting to slowdown, take another week or two off and then switch to routine two and add another rest day. Doing so will make sure that you do not risk overtraining by offsetting the cumulative debt in recovery resources your increasing strength is creating.

(At the beginning of your training program you a literally too weak to overtrain with the weight that you can use on these exercises. However, while your strength grows progressively greater from workout to workout, so too does your ability to create a greater drain upon your recovery reserves increase as well—A 500 pound deadlift imposes a great deal larger drain on the body than a 150 pound one.)

If you find that 10 months or a year into the program your progress stops take one to two weeks off and begin again with one or two more rest days between workouts and/or decrease to an even briefer workout (routine #3). Don't be afraid to increase the rest days between workouts to once every two to three weeks as you progress—remember that in the Haircut Study individuals who performed less exercise less often gained more muscle. Nevertheless, if you make such adjustments along the way you will find that you will make unceasing gains in strength, until you reach your full muscular potential. Once you've reached close to your full potential, the final consolidation routine is your last stop on the road to your full potential.

Routine #3
Workout A
1. Dips—6-10
2. Standing Calve Raise—12-20 (optional)

Workout B
1. Squat—12-20

Workout C
1. Palms-up Pulldown—6-10
2. Military Press—6-10 (optional)

Workout D
1. Deadlift—8-15

And repeat the cycle after workout D.

3. *Pre-Program Considerations:* For all intents and purposes, these routines are perfect. They activate the greatest amount of muscle mass and consume the least amount of your reserve of recovery resources. Yet some individuals may not reap any growth, although highly improbable, yet not impossible, when starting on these programs.

However, since we live in a knowable world of clear-cut certainties, and given that we are dealing with the correct theory of bodybuilding exercise, we come to find that the hindrance of acquiring the desired effect is for the reason that not all of the theory's principles are being appropriately applied. If any given routine is to be productive, it must yield meaningful results immediately; that is to say, you must be getting stronger every workout from commencement to the actualization of your full genetic potential. Since the theory of high intensity training is condensed into three primary principles (intensity, volume, and frequency), one or more of them must not be being applied appropriately.

Volume: Realize that volume consist not merely of the one or three high intensity sets prescribed in the routines, if you are additionally performing unnecessary warm-ups—light sets or cardio—or stretching you are consuming precious energy that can best be used to serve the growth needs of the body.

Frequency: Now understand that when I speak of frequency as a means to recover and overcompensate from the exhaustive effects of the workout I do not exclusively focus on the moment you begin the prescribed training routine. If you were training for months or even years on an overtraining regime, that yielded no results, you have, on basis of obtaining no results, dug a deep, too deep, of a hole in your recovery ability. Recall earlier when I stated that merely three sets of negative only preacher curls required 12 weeks to merely recover from in some instances. Imagine the effects of all of the extensive overtraining you would have done on one of those glorified professional bodybuilder routines!

If you are one of these individuals that has been training unceasingly for the past few months, let alone years, you require time to refill the gigantic hole you have dug in your energy reserves. Take two weeks or even up to two months off, depending on how long you have been overtraining, to fill in the huge deficit you have made in your recovery energies. If you are uncomfortable with taking all of that time off just think of it this way, you haven't gained any muscle with what you have been doing, and since it has been shown that that it can take months for muscle to even to start to atrophy, what do you have to lose? Not muscle, you may even gain some while recovering from your overtraining.

4. *The Importance of Training to Failure:* Some individual will not attain results, even while taking into consideration the recovery needs of their previous training efforts and allowing adequate time between workouts. In this case this individual is not training hard enough, that is, they are not reaching true momentary muscular failure and are merely reaching the point of being uncomfortable or only training until they reach the maximum prescribed repetitions. Remember that it *is* that last seemingly impossible repetition that sets the growth mechanism into motion. I cannot stress enough the importance of

pushing yourself to that last impossible repetition and, even when it seems as if it is impossible, to keep trying to move the weight, even if only by one millimeter. I have had clients that were so determined that at the last repetition, where it seemed as if they were incapable of making the rep, they kept trying with everything they had and, even though it took them well over a minute to finish just the positive phase, they achieved that last rep. It is well worth noting that these were also my clients who *progressed* the greatest.

Perform each exercise to complete momentary muscular failure. Do not terminate a set just because you have reached the maximum recommended number of repetitions prescribed. The most important key component in a workout that is literally responsible for turning on the growth mechanism is effort, not weight. The higher the degree of effort, the high the degree of growth stimulation. Continue until you are unable to continue to positively contract and move the weight no matter how hard you try.

If you desire growth, you are going to have to earn it. Your fundamental temperament during your set should be, "I will get this next rep…even if it kills me." And if you make that nearly impossible rep, you then must become drive to make another. In order for you to stimulate growth, you must attempt the momentarily impossible. Just keep this in mind, you are a volitional being who has the will to fight for a value and push through the extreme discomfort of truly hard work.

5. *Proper Weight Selection and Addition:* If you were to glance at a six and a half foot tall individual weighing 280

pounds and extremely muscular would you consider this individual to be weak or only possessing only an average physical strength? Do you see the huge powerlifters and bodybuilders using one hundred pounds on the squat or only fifty pounds on the bench press?...no, you don't. There *is* an interdependent relationship between strength and size. Consider this, if you were going to develop larger muscles what is going to be the result, you'd get weaker? The name of the game is *progressive overload*, which means, that you must subject your muscles to a greater resistance if they are to grow. Now you realize the fallacy of the untold sums of individuals attempting to workout for muscle size and for muscle strength separately, this is a contradiction (keep in mind Aristotle's law of noncontradictory identification—reality has no contradictions.)

The purpose of every workout performed must be to impose a greater overload in every exercise than the preceding workout. That is, in order to grow bigger and stronger you have to attempt the momentarily impossible. Think of it this way, would you endeavor to improve your vocabulary by repetitively writing and saying your name over and over again? No, in order to improve your vocabulary you would consult a dictionary or a teacher and attempt to pronounce and understand words that are, at the moment, <u>impossible</u> for you.

In order to progress in any endeavor in life you must willing to attempt to perform a given task that you are currently unable to perform, then adapt and grow stronger. Therefore, in reality, a high intensity program is essentially nothing more and nothing less than a strength-training program. The goal is strength...muscle growth is auxiliary, a consequence, a result of the body to the need of greater strength.

For the program I listed above, initial perform 6-10 repetitions for all exercises, except for the squat, leg press, deadlift and calf raise. The reason for the higher repetitions for legs is that over the eons the legs have evolved to tolerate longer bouts of intense activity. The neurons' firing rate in the legs is tremendously distinct from that of the deltoids, arms, chest and back.

If the neurological pathways of the thighs, hips and calves were that of the upper body you would not be able to even walk to the bathroom—try walking on your hands all day, then you'll see the dramatic difference. Neurologically, the thighs, hips and calves are designed for endurance and power—this means more repetitions with very heavy weight. Performing only 6-10 repetitions for the lower body is usually inadequate to activate a high percentage of motor units. Now the reason I prescribe a maximum of 10 repetitions for the upper body and 15-20 for the lower is that we are trying to go to momentary muscular failure, not a long drawn-out process where your lower order muscle fibers are able to recover and be used again.

Now when you start your high intensity, Heavy Duty program do not setoff with reckless abandon when selecting your weight for your exercises. Start off with a weight that has you go to failure within the prescribed range, then after you find your starting weights, assess your training journal with logical evaluation and increase the weight of your exercises when you reach the maximum number of prescribed repetitions. I have made the mistake myself of attempting to increase the weight every workout without considering the fact that my repetitions were at my minimally prescribed range, or lower, the previous workout. As a result, my progress was far less than maximal since I was insufficiently taxing my muscles' capabilities.

Increase the weight of the exercise when you have reached the maximum prescribed repetitions—or beyond—the previous workout by approximately 10 percent to bring you down to the minimum of the rep range.

If you find that your repetitions still increase the next workout, even with a five or ten pound increase, add fifteen or twenty, or even twenty-five pounds the next workout if your repetitions seem too far in excess of ten or more than the range prescribed.

However, if you use so much weight that you find that during your set, you are unable to hold the resistance in the fully contracted position...it is too heavy. Remember that your muscles possess three levels of strength, with positive being the weakest of the three. If you find that you are incapable of holding the resistance once reaching the full contracted position, you did not lift the weight— you threw it!

6. *Rep Modality/High Intensity, Low Force Exercise:* The repetition cadence of every exercise listed, except for the squat and the deadlift, should be of the order of 4-5 seconds for the positive; if there is tension in the fully contracted position (i.e. pulldown and calf raise) pause for 2 seconds; then another 4-5 seconds for the negative portion. If you find that you lift the weight in 3 or 6 seconds and lower it in 3 or 7 seconds, don't worry about

it. The goal is to remove momentum, not distract your focus on the task at hand.

The cadence for the squat and the deadlift should be slightly faster than the others, since while you are in the fully extended position in each of these two exercises it becomes exceedingly hard to breathe properly and to keep proper form. Therefore, these exercises should just be performed with control on the positive, making sure that there is no momentum, and a slower control on the decent. The calf raise should be performed under control, due to the very short range of motion involved, perform the calf raise slow enough that you are under control. The main concern is control and eliminating momentum that turns the exercise into a high force exercise instead of a true high intensity exercise, which is low force and high intensity.

7. *The Importance of Negatives:* Many studies have shown that the most productive portion of the exercise, in terms of muscular size and strength stimulation, is the negative or lower portion of the exercise. In order to gain the greatest benefit from your efforts in the gym you must never avoid the negative by dropping the weight. Aim to obtain the greatest range possible on each exercise by slowly descending from the contracted position into the fully extended position. Such care and focus will not only benefit you muscle growth efforts and prevent risk of injury, but increase your flexibility as well.

8. *Workout Tempo:* Intensity of a workout can also be measured in the amount of work perform within a unit of time. If you were to perform one or two relatively

light warm-up sets for the squat and then set the amount of weight that you thought that you could only get 12 reps with, but instead get 23 gut busting reps before you are unable to get the bar off the safety pins, that would be deemed as true high intensity. However, if you were to take a five or even a fifteen minute rest before you went over to the chin-up bar or dip rack that workout's systemic stimulation would not be of the caliber that would be gained from moving as quickly as possible from exercise to exercise. Yes, you will not, initially, be able to lift as much weight as you could if you were to take a prolonged break between sets, but weight used is not the primary factor in muscular growth stimulation… intensity is the main factor.

Initially you will have to take about two to three minutes before you can mount a dip rack or take hold of the chinning bar without failing because of your cardiovascular conditioning…but that will soon change. I have placed the most demanding exercises first in your routines because, not only because these exercises stimulate the most muscle mass, but due to the repetition range prescribed, they will be the most demanding on your respiratory system. The less time that is taken between sets, the more intense the workout becomes and the greater the stimulus for your body to grow. But do not let your workouts degenerate into a race against the clock and run from exercise to exercise in a semiconscious stagger…take only enough time so you will be able to focus during the next intense set and make the continual effort to gradually lessen the time taken between sets, until you reach the point where you need only the time it takes to quickly walk over to the next exercise and set up the piece of equipment.

Nausea is very common with this very intense type of work so make sure that you carry plenty of water to sip on before the workout, between sets and after the workout... and if you are at the point where you are moving at an appreciable pace between sets, a pail may be necessary. Everyone that I put through this type of intense workout usually spends some time one the carpet...occasionally, but not always, calling for the pail, just incase. But this is to be expected from truly hard work...it is unpleasant, uncomfortable, physically and emotionally demanding... but that only further necessitates the fact that it must be very brief. If you perform this workout in the manner described here you will be finding yourself making excuses to perform *less*...a desire to perform more after you finish the final set is usually a sign that you did not work hard enough. Like I said before, the benefits are yours to reap, but the momentary costs are high.

9. *Save Nothing!:* ...I have found myself coming back to a reoccurring thought of mine. Many individuals that I have trained do not give themselves completely to every set. If they have previously performed a few intense workouts they grasp just how physically and emotionally demanding it can be...so what do they do...they holdback on one or two sets. One major cause for insufficient progress in the efforts of individuals who perform high intensity training is rationalization. They come up with some very self-convincing notion of, "If I don't give everything on this one set and save a little bit for my next set I will get better results on that exercise," or something like, "If I

train at only 80 percent intensity on this set and add one more set of a similar, less demanding, exercise I will get the same result if I were to just go all out on this one."

If you want to get the most out of your time in the gym, you have to give everything you've got on *every single* set. If not, you are just wasting your damn time.... Yes it is unpleasant if done right, yes you will have your subconscious and body screaming at you that you should stop, but if you want to get anywhere, gain anything or reach any higher stair of success in life you have to put forth the requisite effort. I have had young men come up to me, almost drowning in their own damn testosterone, telling me that they are willing do anything and everything to gain larger muscles in the shortest time possible, to which I remember something that I read of Dr. Ken Leistner's, it was something that his father told him, "Some people think they really want something and others really want it." After one or two workouts, many of these individuals that tooted their own horns to the hymn of being an indomitable specimen of true masculinity, suddenly remember imperative business elsewhere and don't return since they say they just do not have time to train anymore…only to find them returning back to gym, performing their volumous routines several times a week that are as intense as pushing pencils. But apparently they just didn't want larger and stronger muscles as much as they thought.

Though many who read this will be tempted by a very power tendency to rationalize the pros of not giving everything they've got every set, just keep in mind that you are only performing one to three exercises, one set each! Save nothing for the next set, forget about the next set completely…your only concern is the set at hand. Then after you reach complete failure, walk over to the next exercise and then center your focus at the task of giving everything you've got on this set.

10. *Training Journal:* As discussed in the previous chapter, it is imperative in your training efforts that you keep a record of your workouts in the gym. Write down all of the exercises that you are doing, the weight you are using, the number of repetitions you achieve and your bodyweight at the *beginning* of each training session.

11. *The Purpose*: The purpose of this program is to facilitate the needs of any individual interested in building muscular size and strength in the most efficacious manner possible. However, if you see that you are genetically predisposed for greater sums of muscle mass and are interested in taking your bodybuilding efforts to the realm of competitive bodybuilding I high recommend that you consult Mike Mentzer's last book *High Intensity Training The Mike Mentzer Way* and *Heavy Duty II: Mind And Body*—which I wholeheartedly contend to be the greatest bodybuilding book written.

12. *Warm-ups:* Some might say at this point, "But you haven't mentioned much about a warm-up or any stretching, and you may hurt yourself if you don't warm-up." Well first of all, you don't need to warm-up the muscles with aerobics or stretching (which has been found to cause more harm than it prevents), because you are not asking that muscle to work hard, at least at the moment you begin the set. The first few repetitions will

actually be a relatively light effort as far as the muscle is concerned, requiring far less force than the muscle is easily capable of producing—thus, in effect, the first few repetitions provide any required degree of a warming-up. Stretching, outside of the stretch provided by full range exercise, only serves to drain upon your body's recovery reserves and adds no benefit.

(Although individual warm-up needs do vary, depending on past injuries, age and room temperature, the only universal prescription for warm-ups I can give is, do the *minimum* amount of exercise you think is required to warm-up the muscles involved in the exercise. If you are going to use warm-up sets at all—remember that the first few repetition serve to further warm the muscles before the last maximum effort rep and that extensive warming up creates an inroad into your adaptive reserves which we are trying to minimize, save for the productive inroad produced from that one set to failure. But if you insist on warming-up at all, I recommend that you only warm-up on the deadlift and the squat as these exercises utilize the largest and greatest number of muscles in the body and will provide for an ample systemic warm-up.)

13. *The Indirect Effect:* As I have mentioned earlier, the biochemical changes that are enacted from the workout take place systemically, throughout the entire body…but there is more to it than that. Heavy, intense exercise has a quite peculiar effect that can be very useful not only in developing bigger muscles, but in rehabilitation of atrophied muscular tissue.

It was in the early 1970's that Arthur Jones noticed what he called "the indirect effect" or "a bilateral effect" of heavy exercise. What Jones was talking about was a unique phenomenon where individuals who would perform heavy and intense exercise for only one side of their body would produce, to a much lesser degree, growth in the other side of their body. Performing, for example, a high intensity set of one-armed nautilus curls for their right arm, over a period of time, and developing a larger left arm to a lesser degree.

What is intriguing about this indirect trend is that the larger the muscle, and quantity of muscles, being put through intense exercise the greater the overall growth of the rest of the body. The squat and deadlift are very special in light of this, as they are the exercises that require the greatest quantity of muscles and the largest muscles of the body, in addition to the capability of utilizing rather prodigious poundage in these movements. In fact, if you were only to perform the squat or deadlift in your workouts for the next year you could possible develop a one or even two-inch increase in the girth of your upper arms...arms that have been abstinent from any really exercise, save for the forearms required for the deadlift.

One aspect of the indirect effect is that the muscles that are closest to the muscle, or muscles, that were made to perform the demanding task appear to receive greater benefit of this growth. So if you were to perform a high intensity set of the leg presses your abdominals, and lower back would receive great levels of indirect growth stimulation, while your upper back and chest would receive lesser degrees of this growth effect, the shoulders receiving a little less, your upper arms receiving even less, and finally your lower arms receiving minimal benefit.

However, the great significance of this phenomenon

is in its practical application to a productive training routine. The goal of a productive workout is to stimulate the greatest amount of muscle mass with the least amount of resources consumed in the process. You will find that the routines listed above follow such guidelines in there *perfect* application—or so close to perfect, that any other modification even possible would be inconsequential in additional efficiency.

14. *Sleep:* Rest is imperative to your progress in the gym. It is during periods of deep sleep that the body's internal environment becomes exceptionally anabolic and undergoes repair. Training with a frequency of once every seven days is far too frequent if you are not allowing your body to rest.... Insomnia is neither the most enjoyable state to be in nor the most productive in terms of recovery…believe me. I have gone months with little more than four to five hours of sleep a night, and say that my progress suffered would be an understatement if I've ever heard one. A proper night's sleep is almost a miracle drug in what it can do for your mental alertness and focus…not to mention the tremendous benefit it has towards your efforts in the gym.

Use commonsense and make the continual effort to get at least eight hours of sleep a night and if you are able to take a nap early in the afternoon, do so. But even resting by relaxing on a couch or lying on the floor while you listen to music or reading a book can be very beneficial to your recovery as well.

Now, one of the stupidest things that I have ever heard…and that is saying something…is the notion of "active rest." There is no such thing as "active" rest…

there is a state of being at rest, either relaxing by reading a book, listening to music or sleeping, and then there is a state of non-rest, where you are performing some type of physical activity. One of the most destructive tendencies of the bodybuilder is the almost inexorable need to do something…because of which, they usually find themselves working out longer or perform long periods of cardio…which eventually leads to a state of being over trained.

The status of a gym rat is not one that should be interchangeable with your name…enjoy your life outside of the gym and do something consonant with your efforts in the gym: study nutrition, study human anatomy, read philosophy and try to grasp the significance of goals in your life, etc. Or reach out into new avenues of study and interest. Make the persistent effort to reach your full human potential both physically and intellectually.

15. *Aerobics:* I will begin this blithe assault on the popular eulogized activity by stating clearly and un-reinterpretable that **I Hate Aerobics!** This detestation is founded upon the gross misunderstandings and outright lies of so-called experts that are respected by literally hundreds of millions of unknowing individuals…experts who end up wasting the lives of countless individuals with grotesque quantities of useless, destructive, endlessly time-consuming, counterproductive exercise.…Prescribed activities that result, in countless cases, with these individuals becoming injured to some extent from such actions. Limiting them with chronic knee, hip, back and ankle pain, to an extent that, if prolonged, will eventually cripple them, possibly

ending in death from the over taxation of one of the many subsystems of the body!

Fundamentally my detestation is not towards the activity itself (though the performance of such a precarious type of activity for health benefits, in light of the fact that proper high intensity training is superior in *every single* aspect of health benefits *infinitely*, is completely asinine—and I am not over exaggerating even slightly…if anything I am underestimating its superiority. How many times can you fit a worth of *zero* into any number?). My detestation is primarily towards the experts whom perform criminal malpractice and have a complete disregard for human life: intentionally avoiding the truth, advocating their subjective beliefs and peer-reviewed traditions in place of reality in a practice where lives are on the line.

The word "Aerobics" is a noun created by Dr. Kenneth Cooper for describing a type of activity: low intensity and high duration (emphasizing running and jogging). The proper scientific term *aerobic*, as he coined the phrase from, is a metabolic energy pathway that requires oxygen to function—utilizing mainly the cardiovascular system.

Dr. Cooper is also the one responsible for popularizing running in North America by correlating it with health—that is, with cardiovascular health (putting emphasis on the conditioning of the heart). And it came to be as of late the 1970's and early 80's, Americans became terrified of the growing rate of heart disease and running caught wind, proliferating into the "craze" that it has now become.

The theory behind Dr. Cooper's stress of "cardiovascular activity" is that the aerobic system requires oxygen to function (as "aerobic" literally means with oxygen) and the key function of the heart is to circulate venous blood through the lungs, picking up oxygen molecules, and circulating oxygen rich blood through the vascular system to supply the tissues that require oxygen to function. And, as Dr. Cooper had learned from his school years, in order for a muscle to improve in its function it must be made to perform work of a demanding nature. However, entangled in the widespread fallacy of equating duration with intensity, Dr. Cooper proclaimed that improving such systems of the body by forcing the heart to perform [over]work of a long and demanding nature would allow greater oxygen uptake and improved heart function. However, as explained in the chapter on overtraining, Dr. Cooper ultimately realized that he had made a gross error in his theory…resulting in a multitude of trainees becoming extremely ill and many were having serious medical problems—like heart disease (the very thing that Dr. Cooper setout to prevent) and cancer.

The heart functions automatically without cognitive exertion, functioning involuntarily 24 hours a day seven days a week for your life. Why should it be necessary to voluntarily (through volitional work of the skeletal muscles) [over]work it to improve its function? "Your pancreas, liver, thyroid and various other organs also function involuntarily every waking moment. Would you ever think to impose added work/stress to improve their function? Would you drink excessive amounts of alcohol to increase the workload on the liver and, thus, improve its function, as exercise specialist, Fred Hahn, once pointed out? No, of course not!" (Mike Mentzer, *Muscle In Minutes*)

What is seldom known, and even less understood, is

that you can only get to the cardiac and vascular systems through the mechanical work of the muscular system. The higher the quality, that is to say the *intensity*, of muscular work, the greater the stimulus for cardiovascular system to improve. The heart, just like all tissues of the body—including the brain—requires a level of intense work that is beyond normal effort to develop. And just like all tissues of the body, when there is a deficit created it requires time to recover and, if the stimulus was sufficient, time to overcompensate. The problem with normal aerobics is that the performance of such activities requires little intensity of effort (lacking an appropriate stimulus for improvement) but a lengthy duration in order to actually tax your cardiovascular system to a sufficient level, but as a result leads to the *overuse* consequences of a retarding agent.

The primary goal for individuals that take-up aerobics is to lose body fat and improve their appearance. The misconception with aerobics by way of fat loss aspirations is that commonly practiced aerobics burn little in the way of calories, in fact, only one pound of fat could sustain ten or more hours of steady state continuous effort. Given that normal Aerobics require few muscle fibers to contract, they burn a miniscule sum of energy. Nonetheless, since most people perform aerobics for long durations and in great frequency, the muscular system is still inordinately taxed, but results in atrophy from overuse. This is why many individuals who perform aerobics day in and day out in an effort to try to lose a few pounds or so look like they have actually gained more body fat and, since their muscular tone has diminished, they take on a "flabby" appearance.

Sadly, when individuals observe that their appearance is not improving they increase the number of days that they run and the number of times they are running a day in an attempt to correct their diminishing physique… only to worsen their state. This leads to loss of self-esteem for many individuals, contemplating their control over existence, questioning if there is something wrong with them…that maybe some people are just not able to achieve their goals, that maybe they possess some idiosyncratic flaw that keeps them from their values that are important to their happiness….No these individuals are not a rare minority of souls, trying to improve their standard of life and failing without answers as to why from the professionals. No…these individuals of sorrow and growing self-doubt seem to be the rule among today's individuals seeking happiness, but going to the wrong source for help.

Know reader that such is not the rule, that there is a reason for everything in the universe, including a lack of bodybuilding/fitness progress—and the reasons are far from infinite. Aerobics, particularly used for the goal of fitness, are counter productive. In fact, many exercise physiologists have semi-realized this and have taken as a step in the right direction for improving cardiovascular condition and caloric burning ability per unit of time. Exercise physiologists and personal trainers are now advocating intense exercise for building muscle as well as conditioning the cardiovascular system, as every pound of additional muscle burns an extra 50-100 calories at rest a day. They alter their recommendations from low intensity, long duration jogging to wind sprints and high intensity interval aerobic training.

Although such takes a great leap into a productive degree of intensity of muscular work, such a manner of exercise is dangerous as hell! Running is one of the most dangerous activities that one can perform, as it subjects the joints to enormous impact force trauma, causing severe damage to the ankles, knees, hips and lower back to a crippling degree...one step forward and two steps back for the scientific community.

The only safe manner to exploit the full potential of the cardiac and vascular systems, as well as one's caloric burning capability, is the performance of high intensity, low force exercise, which is exactly what is prescribed in this book. The efficacy of such training, compared to normal aerobic training was quite prodigiously clarified with a study, funded by Arthur Jones and Nautilus Sports & Medical Industries, conducted at United States Military Academy, West Point in 1975, called Project Total Conditioning. The purpose of the study was to provide the Military Academy with the institutional knowledge of how to use Nautilus exercise equipment properly and to identify the physiological consequences of a high intensity weight training program conducted briefly and infrequently. Researchers sought to answer questions such as: how much skeletal muscle strength can achieved from intense but brief and infrequently exercise, how much does strength training affect an individual's degree of cardiovascular fitness, his degree of flexibility and his overall body composition.

The study involved eighteen cadet football players who trained all of their major muscle groups with ten exercises, one set per exercise three times a week for a period of eight weeks. An extensive battery of tests and measurements were performed on the research group as well as the control group (who just performed regular training practices, jogging, calisthenics and traditional weight lifting without supervision during the study) two weeks into the study and at the conclusion of the eight-week study. The first tests and measurements were two weeks in instead at the beginning because, as Dr. James Peterson wrote in his report of the study, "The pre-study testing was not scheduled until after two weeks of workouts had been completed to minimize the influence of what is commonly referred to as the 'learning effect' on individual performance." And what was the result of only six weeks of high intensity exercise?

After a little less than six weeks of tested training, the eighteen subjects increased the amount of weight that they could use in the ten exercises by 60 percent! In addition to this, despite such a tremendous increase in their strength and the weight that they were using, their workout time actually dropped to a mere nine minutes a session of actual training towards the end of the eight-week experiment.

As a measure of the functional application of high intensity training the research group, as well as the control group, were administered three tests: a two-mile run, the 40-yard dash and a vertical jump. With the two-mile run, the test subjects' improvement was 4.32 times greater than the control group, 4.57 times greater in the 40-yard dash and close to two times greater in the vertical jump. What about cardiovascular improvement? During the testing periods, the cardiovascular testing was conducted by Arthur Jones' people, the West Point researchers, a number of outside experts and even Dr.

Coopers own people…the results? Well the cardiovascular improvement in the test subjects was so great that Dr. Cooper refused to believe them, even though his own people did all of the pre and post-testing.

How good were the results? Well that the beginning of the second week, when the first functional test was performed, the test subjects required approximately forty minutes to complete the workout and there heart rate was at a continuous surplus of 210 beats per minute, that was sustained for forty minutes. After six weeks the subjects were tested again, only it did not require the same amount of time, they completed the workout in only thirty minutes with 60 percent more weight. In addition to this, their heart rates never reached above 192, even though Arthur Jones' people were leaning on them to move faster between exercises and push harder.

With regards to flexibility, the crowd of experts tested the test subjects and the control group with four measures of flexibility: trunk flexion, trunk extension, shoulder flexion and shoulder extension. The test subjects achieved a much higher degree of improvement of flexibility than the control group. In fact, they averaged an 11 percent increase in flexibility while the control group members only averaged a 0.85 percent increase!

Earlier I mentioned how many exercise physiologists publish falsified research studies that usually cannot be trusted at face value. So why do I believe this study? Well this study, funded by Arthur Jones at a cost of $1,000,000.00, had a few things that most exercise physiologists do not offer. Arthur Jones had many experts from around the country and even biased enemies in business perform the tests; the West Point Military Academy, full of some of the most trustworthy and honest individuals in the country, who can testify to the validity of the study; in addition to a large part of the $1,000,000.00 in expenses incurred by Nautilus resulted from having recorded the entire study on 16mm professional motion picture film using more than a dozen professional cameras. In the words of Arthur Jones, "All together we used more than 500,000 feet of film. All of these cameras being synchronous, meaning that the film was exposed at an exact rate of 24 frames per second, thereby providing us with an exact record of the time involved in each exercise, speed-of-movement used during the exercise as well as time elapsed." The most important factor that proves beyond a shadow of a doubt the validity of this study is that, unlike most purported studies, this test is objectively demonstrable, i.e., these type of results are repeatable no matter who performs the test.

How volitionally blind or just plain inept are many of today's experts you might ask? Well in a 2006 radio interview, a certain Dr. who will not be mentioned (who is one of today's most well known exercise physiologists) stated that he has never seen any research proving that one set of high intensity exercise will do anything for an increase in muscular size and strength. He states that with multiple metanalyses—a highly inaccurate and problematic method of research that is diluted with innumerable non-sensible and false research—that there is not enough proof of the productiveness of one set to failure...after which he goes on to say that by standing on a vibrating platform that violently shakes the hell out of you, you will somehow increase muscle strength and muscle mass....It becomes quite astonishingly clear the stupidity of today's self-stylized experts when they are faced with such practically evident-truths and fight them, turning to the ridiculous and proclaiming that this "new thing" that they supposedly discovered, yet is usually a previous scam of the past that has been forgotten enough to use again with a new title, is the answer....But they never really explain why or having any proof as to how.

Someone once said that, "figures don't lie, but liars always figure"...but in the field of exercise a more valid, and sadly more accurate, statement would be, "figures are almost always based on lie and liars created these figures."

However, as my research and personal training goes on, I realize more and more, almost everyday, the accuracy of something that Arthur Jones use to say, "There are two types of people in the world: the ignorant and the stupid. We are all inherently ignorant...ignorance means lacking knowledge. Ignorance is correctable, with effort you can gain knowledge of what you are ignorant of... stupidity, those who choose to avoid reason when faced with undeniable facts and proof. Well...that seems to be genetic and permanent!"

Aerobic activity is popularly synonymous with "fitness" and "health," as in, the performance of aerobics is going to make you more physically fit and better your health. Well this assumption is completely contradictory to the truth. If your goal is to condition your aerobic system, you are better off doing it in the most effective and efficient manner possible. The simple fact is that properly performed high intensity training will train *every* metabolic system of your body, especially your aerobic system. The aerobic system *serves to support the muscular system* and if the muscular system is to improve, your aerobic system must follow suit. A better way to explain this is by imagining that your skeletal muscular system possesses 100 units of functional ability and your other metabolic systems have 100 units of functional ability. Now let us say that by some magical spell you increase your muscles functional ability to 200 units or, for a dramatic demonstration, 100,000 units. However, your other metabolic systems only possess 100 units of functional ability…what is your body's overall functional ability? It is still only 100 units.

If the body lacks the metabolic support for its potential strength it is limited to the maximum ability of the other metabolic systems, so it only makes sense that if your body's muscular functional ability is to improve, all systems that support it are to do the same.

High intensity training has unfortunately be misinterpreted as purely "anaerobic" exercise, not aerobic—but this is not so. As Dr. Doug McGuff pointed out, high intensity training is a "Global Metabolic Conditioning" form of exercise that involves and conditions all metabolic systems of the body, anaerobic and aerobic.

Does all of this information summed up mean that aerobics or any additional physical activity outside of your high intensity program is completely useless, needing to be avoided at all costs? Absolutely not! The purpose of high intensity training is to improve your physical condition to allow you to perform more successfully in the activities you enjoy in life and improve your physique's muscular prowess and attractiveness. If you were to abdicate all the activities you enjoy in life, whether it be rock climbing, hockey, swimming or anything else, you would, as Dr. Doug McGuff put it, be giving someone a Ferrari and telling them to only to drive it in a school zone. Remember, bodybuilding is meant to enhance your life, not to consume it! If you truly enjoy the activity and are not merely using it for "supposed" health benefits, go for it. Just take your additional physical activity into consideration when gauging your recovery needs of your bodybuilding program.

16. *The Abdominals*: The abdominals, for the most part, do not articulate around a single joint. They articulate around a multifaceted joint in a sort contractile stroke. In order to fully contract the abdominals you need merely contract your stomach a few inches by depressing your rib cage and/or by elevating your pelvis. When performing the underhand pulldown and the squat your abdominals are statically engaged in "stabilization." This concept of being used for stabilization branches off into two major misconceptions.

Firstly, most fitness minded individuals believe that the abdominals are solely stabilizer muscles. This simply is not true. The abdominal muscles function in the same manner as all of your skeletal muscles: isometrically and dynamically. All of skeletal musculature is capable of contracting dynamically, moving through a given range of motion, and isometrically, by holding one position statically. All muscles, in a sense, can be "stabilizers." However, this does not elicit a different method to train them; it merely demonstrates a muscular function that can be trained more efficiently through direct and intense contractions instead of a stability ball or training on an unbalance surface...all of which are inefficient in stimulating the abdominals, in addition to being outright dangerous.

The second misconception is that you need to train the abdominals specifically with crunches and sit-ups in order to develop them. This misconception has allowed a multi-million dollar "ab-fitness" industry to emerge, since Americans are infatuated with their abs and willing to try almost anything to produce the à la mode "six-pack." The truth is that the abdominals are engaged in almost every exercise you perform whether you know it or not, and with the underhand pulldown and squat they are significantly loaded and will be very effectively stimulated, allowing all the incentive needed to develop your abdominal musculature.

17. *Equipment*: In performing any of the preceding exercises, I highly suggest the use of exercise machines with a guided range of motion. The reason for this is that through high intensity training your aim is to increase your strength, not to develop the *skill* to lift a barbell correctly. With an exercise machine with a guided motion, like a smith machine or Nautilus pullover, the only focus of the trainee is lifting the weight, that's it.

When using a barbell or any free roaming piece of equipment your strength in that exercise is heavily contingent on your skill in the movement. When performing a barbell bench press for instance, you need to develop the skill of the *specific* balance required to move the barbell through a particular groove. If you did not follow the groove and merely press the barbell in a straight line, you would be moving the barbell straight over your genitals. Remember, the goal of a high intensity workout is to only overload the muscles and not to additionally encumber your neurological system with trying to develop a specific skill. If however your goal is to become a competitive powerlifter, this skill requires development.

If you have access to Nautilus (1st or 2nd generation or 2ST are the only ones I recommend), MedX (both the selectorized and their plate-loaded counterpart Avenger) or Hammer Strength equipment, use them instead of free weights. All of these machines have guidance moment arms that follow as closely as possible to muscular and joint function. They also possess a cam and/or leverage curve that varies the resistance as to follow the strength curve of the particular muscles being employed. Use of these machines will enhance your muscular progress and significantly increase the safety of your workout.

If you do not have access to these machines a regular barbell in a power rack of some sort, having safety pins in, as to avoid possible injury, is still extremely efficacious in stimulating tremendous muscle growth. However, I highly suggest that you use these machines if you can instead of free weights for safety and being able to purely focus on the lift and not balancing the bar. Additionally, free weights do not vary the resistance in accordance with muscular and joint function, so you will inevitably reach a sticking point in the exercise that is considerably harder than any other position—the equipment listed about will not delimit you because of strength curve incompatibility. But if you are devoid of these machines designed with scientific precision, a barbell, a set of dumbbell, a chin-up bar and a dip rack are, more often than not, more beneficial that most exercise equipment companies out there. But whatever you use, whether it is a rusty barbell or a five thousand dollar MedX machine, the only factors that decide whether you stimulate muscle growth or not is the intensity of effort and a progressive increase in weight used, not the specific equipment of use.

18. *What is Possible*: So what kind of progress can one expect to gain from high intensity training? This is an extremely difficult question to answer, since we currently do not possess the technology to accurately assess an individual's full genetic potential beyond a rough estimation of some of the more ostensive muscle potential factors—such as muscle belly length, skeletal structure and an predisposition to being more muscular than average—and muscular biopsies used to analyze myostatin levels and other proteins that detail your catabolic/anabolic profile.

Yes, you can expect continuous and worthwhile results from the beginning of your program to your full physiologic potential. However, what kind of progress is dependent on your genetics and your intensity. Nevertheless, if you pay your dues in the gym...the rewards are tremendous by any standard.

Diamonds the size of basketballs!—Results? I have had one beginner increase the functional ability of their hip and thigh muscles to such a degree that their performance on the leg press went from 20 reps with 105 pounds to 50 reps with 320 pounds in under two months! I have had another individual start out at a 50 pound deadlift, and in two months of training—performing the deadlift every other week—he became so strong that he was using well over 300 pounds! That is a strength increase in excess of 600 percent! Such results are not abnormal, but typical to the average gains from high intensity training. One individual that I was training gained 21 pounds of muscle in only four workouts, while I had another individual gain an equally impressive improvement of 15 pounds of muscle in three months on a relatively small frame.

The results of most individuals reaching their full genetic potential are an average of 30 pounds of muscle. At this moment, some reading this will notice that this is not the amount of muscle that they hoped for…maybe even becoming disappointed at such low prospects. However, if you are dissatisfied with such a likely genetic possibility, go to your local grocery store and walk over to the meat section. Look for one pound of beef steak, hold it in you hands and try and gather twenty-nine more and image all of those slabs of meat deposited all over your body. That is a hell of a lot of tissue! That is enough muscle to make the average 155 pound male look like a Herculean John Grimek or Frank Zane.

It should also be known that out of that 155 pounds of bodyweight only about 20 pounds is muscle (the rest being bone, water, fat, waste materials and inorganic matter). Therefore, if the 155 pound average American male were to gain 30 pounds of *pure* muscle (as opposed to 30 pounds of bodyweight that is a varying composition of fat and muscle) he would literally transform his body by more than doubling his existing muscle mass!

There might even be a chance that you possess the kind of genetic potential of Sean Robertson, who was a former client of Mike Mentzer. In only a four-year period, Sean went from a sickly thin bodyweight of 125 pounds at a height of 5 feet 6 inches, to an unbelievable muscular bodyweight of 250 pounds!

What are you capable of gaining? No, most individuals reading this will not have the rare genetic make-up to become a champion physique athlete or professional sports athlete, such genetic anomalies are very few and far between. This does not mean that you cannot enjoy trying to compete in bodybuilding competitions or athletic competitions, you may actually become quite good at them, even having an advantage over some genetically superior athletes by intellectual, logical guidance to improve your body more efficiently. But do not dwell on short muscle bellies or a poor skeletal frame; take pride in your capability of improving your situation, in your ability to realize a genetic potential with rational thought and prolific motivation. Sean Robertson was not heavily muscled from the start nor was former world champion bodybuilder Roy Callendar, who looked like an Auschwitz victim before he started training. But you will never know what your potential is unless you try to develop your body to its full potential through the most efficacious manner possible. With a properly conducted high intensity training program many trainees will be able to actualize their full genetic potential in one year or less.

19. *Fundamentals of Nutrition:* The fundamental requirements of nutrition are actually quite simple to understand. However, with the frame of mind held by today's health fanatics, they embark upon problems of the sorts that are equivalent to algebra and calculus when they lack the fundamental understanding of addition and

subtraction. Searching high and lower for the secret vile or lotion that will bring them all that they desire without the discomfort of either intellectual deliberation or physical effort. Supplements, herbs, "organic" produce, "miracle diets," and items of the like are the popular trend today because if it.

An intense, concise, perusal of the biological needs of the body reveals a universal definition of all areas of nutritional needs. The most precise and the clear-cut method of describing the scientific definition of nutrition is by the single solitaire word that has great significance in the sciences of biology, sociology, economics and psychology: *Need*. This word "need" concerns your body's specific need for certain nutrients in a specific quantity.

If you have ever taken biology or a nutritional course you would recognize that the concept need, when applied to nutrition, implies a set limit that cannot be transcended. An organism's nutritional need is a set point, for which anything imposed over what is needed is simple disposed of or stored (to a certain capacity) and going over this point will not force the body to utilize more of it nor increase the functional ability of the substance's intended biological purpose. It may actually become harmful, as researchers have found that under certain circumstances, such as when vitamins are consumed in excess, it might actually promote the production of free radicals and displace other biologically active compounds from storage.

So now the intelligent question arises, what exactly does the body need and why? Realize that never in the history of mankind has man had such a plethora of myriad possibilities with his food. But where does one obtain his nutritional needs in an ocean, rife with selection?

In order to maintain good health (a first requisite to muscle growth) and provide for optimal growth, our bodies require more than 40 different primary nutrients and hundreds of plant compounds. These various nutrients can be found in the six primary food components: water, carbohydrates, proteins, fats, vitamins and minerals.

Water: Amidst a provocative symphony of enzymes, inorganic matter and histological substrates lays a medium that is the founding requisite for all life…water. Though the main physiologic construct of all muscular tissue comprises of protein, the dominate substance within a muscle's composition is not protein, but water. Muscle is actually more than 70 percent water. The human body itself is comprised of two-thirds water, which accounts for the fluidity of your blood and lymph system.

Water is our waste remover through elimination of urine and feces; it lubricates the joints; keeps our body temperature within a very narrow margin; allows the kidneys and liver to function properly in breaking down lipids; and last, but not least to the bodybuilder, water is the primary constituent of muscle tissue. Viewed with the proper attention it deserves, water is the most important nutrient for survival and growth. Water allows the removal of the metabolic byproducts produced by your workouts and the transportation of anabolic hormones to the muscle cell's hormone receptors—adequate hydration actually increases the exposure of these hormonal receptor sites to the flood of anabolic hormones stimulated by the workout.

But while it is true that our muscles are most

comprised of water and adequate hydration sustainably enhances recovery and anabolic hormonal pickup, it does not follow that we should drink gallons of it a day to increase muscle growth. Water, like all nutrients, is toxic if consumed in extreme excesses. Water plays a very crucial role in the balance of electrolytes in the body. An over consumption of water to an extreme degree can disturb your electrolyte balance and disrupt the cardio-rhythmic function of your heart. So while water is of great importance, it is not the only important nutrient. Just use commonsense with your water intake and make a decent effort to take-in an appropriate amount of water with the goal of consuming approximately 2-3 liters a day.

Carbohydrates: Ah yes, carbohydrates. In Western society, this macronutrient has lost its once worshipped luster and has been condemned for its misconceptions and misuses. Such a mistress of sin and lust among individuals of the fad diet genre—people who helplessly give into the naughty indulges of cake and ice cream under the twilight swaying through the translucent fabric of the curtains over the kitchen window. Stewing in a torrent of ecstasy, as the simple moment of such indescribable pleasure, binging brought about by a low or zero carbohydrate intake, blanks-out all of the feared consequences of this crime in intimate affairs.

Carbohydrates, as I mentioned above, are a macronutrient in a group containing three others: Fat, Alcohol and Protein. The group is called Macro for a particular reason: they are all needed in great quantities, save for alcohol, as they are the only nutrients that provide energy. The need of this so-called "fattening" substance is essential for normal function of one's body and mind.

Carbohydrates are the primary fuel source for the brain, the muscles, the immune and nervous systems. Carbohydrate depletion affects not only the duration and intensity of physical exertion but also coordination, reaction time, and mental focus. This is quite readily available to understand, as the brain is comprised of approximately 80 percent of a substance called Glia cells, for which *their main function is to store sugar*. The brain in fact derives approximately 99.9 percent of its nutrients from sugar.

Carbohydrates are the preferred source of fuel for the body. But all of the four macronutrients contain different quantities of calories (energy) that can be used: protein yields four calories per gram, carbohydrates hold four calories per gram, alcohol holds seven calories, and fat has nine calories per gram. The substitution of protein, fat or alcohol as the main contributors to the caloric intake of a diet can come with some serious health risks: high protein diets tax the kidneys and liver and can cause irreparable damage, and there have even been numerous reported deaths since the 1970's caused by extremely high protein diets; high fat diets, specifically high in saturated and trans fats, cause risk of heart and colon disease; high alcohol diets can cause multiply health problems that need not be listed—examples are everywhere nowadays.

Since your main concern as a bodybuilder is to build bigger and stronger muscles, you require the proper energy to fuel intense bouts of exercise. The body stores glucose (simplified sugar) in the muscles and liver as a glucose polymer called glycogen. A high intensity workout utilizes predominately glucose to fuel the demands of the muscles. If you want to stimulate muscle growth to the greatest degree you are going to have to put in premium fuel instead of a dirty fuel that is synthesized from fat and protein in the food you eat or broken-down and synthesized from your muscles—a fuel that can potentially be harmful to the machine (the body).

The bottom line comes down to the fact that you should consume ample amounts of carbohydrates in your diet and not limit yourself to bran products for carbohydrates—a candy bar once in a while won't do any harm, as long as it is in moderation. A proper diet for normal health, athletic and bodybuilding needs should be constituted of approximately 40-50 percent of the calories you consume being carbohydrates from carbohydrate rich foods, such as, fresh fruits and vegetables, and cereals and grains.

Protein: Protein constitutes approximately 22 percent of muscular tissue and is the main building block of life. This however has been overemphasized in our culture today, as fitness minded individuals, athletes and bodybuilders alike dive into the notion that, "Since my muscle tissue is composed of protein, it only makes sense that more protein equals more muscle."

Understand that these individuals are basing there muscle building philosophy on the simplistic faith in more is better. To finally put this philosophical premise to rest I will state that the more is better philosophy can only be only conceivably valid in two circumstances: money and girls...and even these two are questionable.

The fallacy of this idea can quickly be demonstrated in an extreme hypothetical situation: say that you start drinking water and never stop. The idea is that, since you body composition consists of mostly water, consuming more will make you bigger, stronger, and more efficient. You quickly realize that this notion is erroneous, as you soon become water logged or even sick. However, with that "can do" attitude that those motivational tapes bestowed upon you—telling you that all of your little problems are just in your head—you continue on with persistent consumption, striving for greater and greater hydration! But with one last gulp you either drown or you dilute the electrolytes of you body and disturb the cardio-rhythmic function of your heart…and you die.

In the case of protein, it possesses the same molecular structure as carbohydrates and fat, but with an additional molecule: nitrogen. This nitrogen molecule is needed by the body, but with an over consumption, resulting from high protein diets, the body becomes incapable of properly utilizing it, so it attempts to secrete it. This process requires a great amount of work from the liver and kidneys (which may cause hypertrophy and severe irreparable damage). The body will need excess amounts of water in order to excrete the nitrogen as well. This might cause dehydration, as the body will extract fluids from the organs and muscular tissues in order to accomplish the task.

In a proper diet, your protein consumption should contribute around 25-35 percent of your daily calories. This is all that is *needed* to allow for the repair and construction of more muscle tissue. If anything, I have recommended too much…but that is debatable.

Fats: Fats, to quote Mike Mentzer, are not the bogeyman that so many make them out to be, as fats sheath the nerves, synthesis many enzymes, allow for the production of many anabolic hormones, can aid in increasing insulin sensitivity and help proper digestion. In addition to this, certain vitamins are fat soluble...so obviously fats play a crucial role in a well-balanced diet.

Fat are divided into saturated and unsaturated fats. Saturated fats are found in animal products and are solid at room temperature. Many studies have shown that high saturated fat intake can lead to heart problems. Unsaturated fats, most notably Omega-3, which are mostly found in plants, olive oils and nuts, have been shown to have multiple health benefits from preventing cancer and heart disease to assisting the promotion of fat loss and a positive anabolic hormonal profile. We would do well to limit our saturated and try to eliminate trans fat consumption in a proper diet, but it would also be highly advantageous to the bodybuilder to increase his consumption of unsaturated fats. I recommended a dietary intake of 15-35 percent fat. But attempt to acquire these fats from nuts, olives, avocados, olive oils, green leafy vegetables and fish.

Vitamins & Minerals: All of the various vitamins and minerals are referred to as micronutrients, since they are needed only in small amounts. Recommended dietary intake for vitamins and minerals is measured in milligrams as opposed to the grams used for the macronutrients. Vitamins and minerals combine in the body to form the enzymes that function as catalysts in innumerable important physiological processes.

If you consume at least a reasonably well balanced, you are acquiring all the vitamins and minerals you need. Our daily needs for the micronutrients are quite small, so don't waste your time consuming handfuls of pills thinking that your body will utilize them. Most will pass off through urination—only making your urine very expensive—, while some vitamins, especially the fat-soluble ones, become toxic in large doses.

* * *

Your primary concern for acquiring an optimal diet—that which supplies the body with all of its biological needs—should be to obtain a well-balanced diet on a daily basis, consisting of a diverse plethora of different foods. A balanced diet requires no supplements nor "special" foods nor herbal medicine. The notion that man can only live a "healthy life" through supplemental dietary habits is grotesque and far from true. Man has survived for millions of years without the implementation of extreme quantities of additional nutrient consumption. If such were the case…if man honestly required, by nature, the consumption of immense quantities of vitamins and minerals…mankind would have never made it out of the womb.

A balanced diet will result in sublime improvement in performance ability in athletes, dieters and average none goal-oriented individuals who have been following one of the many ridiculous diets espoused by experts who try to get their name out in the world by making up their own "original miracle" diet.

A well-balanced diet, by definition, is one that satisfies *all* of your nutritional needs, the makeup of a balanced diet is the consumption of the four basic food groups: fruits and vegetables, cereals and grains, meat and high-protein products, and milk and dairy products.

1. Fruits and Vegetables: Fruits and vegetables are very nutritious and will supply your body with a plethora of vitamins, minerals, flavonoids, phytochemicals and polyphenols (which have been shown to have great antioxidant potential with anti-cancer and heart disease prevention qualities). They also provide the bulk of cellulose fiber that is crucial for elimination and keeping your gut healthy. An intake of six or more servings a day is recommended.

2. Cereal and Grain Foods: Baked goods, oats, bread and flour products are a rich, but cheap in cost, source of carbohydrates, minerals, and protein. They also contribute little to your saturated fat intake. This group will be the main contributor to your important carbohydrate intake, so bodybuilders must not skimp on their consumption of cereals and grains. An intake of four or more servings a day is recommended.

3. The Meat and High-protein Group: This group includes fish, beef, eggs, poultry, dried beans, nuts and peas. This group will be the main contributor to protein in your diet and provides essential B vitamins and iron. Three or more servings a day is recommended. (A basic serving of meat is approximately 3.5 ounces)

4. Milk and dairy products: Milk and other dairy products are a very rich source of protein, calcium and riboflavin. Try to consume reduced fat milk products like skim and non-fat milk if you can, as regular milk products possess a high number of calories. Two or more servings a day is recommended.

* * *

With a balanced diet you are acquiring all of the nutrients that your body requires...it really is that simple. For some, if not most, individuals, this diet will be occasionally supplemented...but not with vitamins, minerals or protein supplements, but with luxury foodstuffs, such as chocolates, sweets, butter, etc. And this is still sensible, if taken within reason, in the commitment to a proper healthy diet.

9

Supplementary Concerns

During periods of progress (i.e. during muscle size and strength increases), one's physiology is not still, but in a constant state of fluctuation. It is astounding how many bodybuilders today still do not understand the requirement of increasing strength in order to increase muscular size. Size increase is a corollary of a strength increase. When one does grasp this physiologic absolute and regulates their program to accommodate their required recovery needs from intense bouts of exercise, permitting enough time between workouts to become stronger every workout, it is only then that nutrition becomes a factor in their bodybuilding efforts. Realize that it is *only* in the context of having employed the proper training method that nutrition becomes a consideration.

(Even if the muscle promoting supplements that are espoused by the bodybuilding orthodoxy did "enhance" muscle growth, they are inert without a stimulus that turns on the body's growth mechanism. And even when nutrition becomes a fact in your bodybuilding progress, it is actually quite simple; it is really just basic common sense: make a reasonable effort to consume a well-balanced diet everyday, rich in plenty of fruits, vegetables and lean meats.)

You will grow stronger each workout following the workout program listed in the previous chapter. However, when an individual grows stronger week-to-week it is evident that there is a continuous physiologic change happening inside their muscles. Since a given muscle only has the potential of contracting with a certain amount of force that is dependent on its cross-sectional area, a muscle that is continuously growing stronger cannot be the same muscle workout to workout. If the muscle did not change, it would be limited to the identical amount of contractile capability as it was the previous workout.

If during this period of change, a bodybuilder only acquires a maintenance caloric intake (i.e. only consuming enough calories to maintain their current bodyweight) they will, by the laws of physics, or more precisely thermodynamics, maintain only their current level of mass. However, it has been demonstrated by the Haircut study, the research of John Little and Arthur Jones that one can gain muscle while on a maintenance intake or even a caloric deficit.

A paradox? No, this is not a metaphysical contradiction percolating through the sea of causality, but a complex internal biologic alteration of energy and matter between muscular and adipose tissues. Remember, muscle tissue is constituted mostly of water and its total mass is less than a quarter protein. As a result, as long as one consumes a balanced diet rich in carbohydrates with sufficient amounts of protein and a regular water intake, the body can literally "steal" substrates from fat and use them to assist the growth of muscular tissue.

However, though this is possible, I have noticed with my clients and personal experience that this ability is also a genetically mitigated physiologic trait that will have some individuals being able to gain remarkable amounts of muscular size and lose fat at an equally astonishing rate, contrasted with individuals who can barely, if at all, gain muscle and loss fat at the same time. In addition to this, I have found that there is a sort of "physiologic wall" for this trait. The human body is a survival organism and its first and foremost priority is its own survival. If you are asking the body to create more of the body's most metabolically expensive tissue, without the consumption of calories required for its sustainment, it will do everything possible to prevent an increase in muscle mass.

For that reason, if you are to actualize the full potential of the muscle mass stimulated by the workout, a caloric surplus is necessary to optimize a muscular surplus. The body will not sustain continual muscular size progression without the nutritional stimulus indicating to the body that it has caloric energy and matter available to fulfill the increasing caloric demand of additional muscular tissue. Gaining muscle on a caloric deficit is less than optimal and progressively deteriorates in the rate of muscular size and strength increases; however, a wild consumption of indiscriminate sums of calories will only lead you to getting fat. If you are to do this scientifically, you have to make the effort of acquiring a baseline, understanding your body's current caloric needs.

To do this you need to discover your daily caloric needs. You can do this by simply recording everything you eat and drink, along with the quantity that you consumed that day in a food diary (note: a nutritional scale that is preprogrammed with the caloric value of foods can be indispensable in your fat loss and muscle gaining efforts, but a regular food scale is very effective as well). A food diary will help you control and scientifically analyze your diet, allowing you to keep your intake and the caloric values of different foods in perspective of your goals—doing so after a few weeks will allow you to roughly estimate the calories of certain foods based on their portion size…making life a lot easier than it would be if you were to try and calculate the caloric value of everything you ate for the rest of your life. At the end of the day sit down with a calorie counting book or a nutritional calorie counting website and tally up that day's caloric total. Continue doing this for the next 7 days and at the end of day 7, if your body weight did not change, add together all the calories consumed for a weekly total and divide it by seven and you will have your daily caloric maintenance level.

So from here let us say, hypothetically, that your daily maintenance of calories is 2500. Upon embarking on the routine listed in the previous chapter, you could expect to make a very incredible gain of about 30 pounds of muscle in a year for the average beginner. Now let us analyze how many additional calories a day are required to facilitate such tremendous growth. Since one pound of muscle equals 600 calories, we multiply that by 30 to get 18,000 calories on top of your maintenance caloric need. So how many additional calories do you need to consume a day to facilitate such growth? Well since you need an additional 18,000 in a *year's time,* we divide 18,000 by 365 days in a year to determine that you require only 50 additional calories above your maintenance level a day… such only seems to make bodybuilders who consume hundreds and hundreds of extra calories a day, only to gain 30 to 50 pounds of fat in the off session, trying to "bulk-up," look quite ridiculous.

To try to optimize your muscle growth by consuming thousands of indiscriminate sums of calories in an effort to "bulk-up" is just worse than a waste of your time. Worse because once you've gained the muscle you wanted, it takes a long time, and a lot of discomfort, to lose all of the fat that you will gain, potentially requiring you to sacrifice some of that hard-earned muscle in the process. So in concert with the high intensity program described in the previous chapter, make a daily effort to consume a surplus of 50 to 100 calories above your maintenance level. Doing so makes sure that you are consuming enough calories to provide the requisite substrates and energy needed for additional muscle growth.

(Logically analyzing the degree of your strength increases will serve as a relative indicator of how much growth was stimulated. If you are only increasing a rep or two and increasing the weight here and there and if you are scrupulously monitoring your recovery needs— inserting additional recovery days when progress begins to slow and taking a week or two off every 3-4 months or so—, obviously there is less growth stimulation than if you were improving by five or so reps and/or increasing the weights used a workout by 20 or more pounds.)

Now, a caloric surplus of 50 to 100 is a reasonable recommendation that should serve the needs of your body's growth mechanism, however, some individuals might gain some fat as well. The surplus I prescribe is an ample amount that might add minute amounts of body fat for some individuals. But do not fret. One pound of fat requires 3500 calories. And even with individuals that only require 16 calories surplus for muscle growth and the other 84 calories would turn to fat, in a month, only three quarters of a pound of fat would be gained. However, do not despair, with the possession of a larger sum of muscle mass you will have raised your basal metabolic rate and increased you ability to burn calories while doing nothing, thus, you will be able to lose body fat with less discomfort of lessening food consumption.

However, just because your body may only require 16 additional calories a day to produce muscular tissue it does not mean that the rest of the calories are stored as fat. The human body, as all machines—whether organic or mechanic—that perform mechanical work, is not 100 percent efficient with the energy it consumption. Automobiles possess a thermal efficiency of around 21 percent and electric power plants have a thermal efficiency of around 13 percent. This means that out of all the energy put in, only a small percent is actually utilized for the intended function. The human body has an approximate efficiency of 25 percent. This means that out of the total sum of calories required to perform metabolic and mechanical work only a quarter of it is actually utilized for its intended purpose. The byproduct of this inefficiency is heat, as noticed when you perform a heavy set of squats or deadlifts in a cool room and afterwards you are perspiring profusely. Creating new tissue is an extremely demanding task for your body that requires time and energy, so you may find that a caloric surplus of 50-100 is just perfect for your bodybuilding efforts.

If you find however that while on a surplus of 100 calories a day your bodyweight remains the same for a period of months (judging by a day to day or even a week to week basis is erroneous, as something like a 10 pound increase of muscle a year will not register a change in weight day to day or week to week—normal scales are just not sensitive enough to pickup such small variations), bump your daily intake another 100 or 150 calories and you should see your weight begin to increase, but be careful. Remember that your goal is to serve the needs of the growth mechanism and not to "bulk up" as many professional bodybuilders do. An indiscriminate consumption of additional calories will not promote further muscle growth, but it does place stress on the body. Synthesizing triglycerides at an extraordinary rate places a huge total on the body's systemic recovery resources. As a result, overly excessive food consumption will interfere with the function of the body's growth mechanism and will impede your muscular gains.

A Word on Fat Loss

With your daily caloric needs established, you possess the requisite knowledge to start losing fat. Simply reduce your caloric intake by 500-750 calories a day from your maintenance level. But never allow your daily intake to go below 1300 calories for males and 1000 for females, as below this you are unable to obtain a balanced diet and are at risk of muscle catabolism. With this recommendation, you can expect a weekly loss of 1 to 1.5 pounds of fat a week.

However, if you were to attempt to lose body fat without the physiologic stimulus of a high intensity workout—telling your body that it its current level of muscle mass, bone density, connective and nervous tissues are required, or that it needs more of them, to deal with the threat of the workout—your body will make the executive decision to remove some body fat and some muscle, bone, connective and nerve tissue.

If you desire substantial results, the performance of a high intensity workout once every 7 to 21 days will build muscular tissue that will increase your metabolism and thus increase your caloric burning capability, as well as increase bone mineral density, connective tissue strength and increase nervous tissue. The workout, due to your lower caloric intake, should be vastly reduced in both volume and frequency, as you lack the needed calories to fuel and recover from longer duration workouts. However, since the proscribed program is of the lowest volume it serves both as the ultimate muscle building routine in addition to the definitive fat loss program—a study conducted at Nautilus North, by John Little and Cary Howe, found that by performing only one set a workout produced substantial greater results that two sets when in concert with a caloric deficit.

So if you decide to begin a caloric deficit diet to loss excess body fat and get cut, reduce your workouts to one-two sets a workout. A routine that stimulates all of the major muscle groups over a three-workout period (routine #3) is listed in the previous chapter. This routine will allow you to stimulate the greatest amount of muscle mass with the absolute least amount of resources consumed, allowing you to progress in both muscle growth and fat loss for approximately 12 weeks of dieting.

Dieting for longer than 12 weeks, unless you are obese and are prescribed by a physician to maintain a longer period of dieting, may have some negative health effects, in addition to negatively affecting your muscle gains. After you reach your goal in leanness, simply add approximately five hundred calories to your diet.

So how much can you expect to lose on such a program? For the average non-over fat individual, a loss of 1 to 2 pounds *maximum* a week is healthy, as more could be a sign of a caloric intake that is far to low.

(The truth is that it is physiologically impossible for anyone to lose one pound of body fat a day under normal circumstances. Any diet or exercise program that produces weight loss—not fat loss—of one pound a day or more is relying on a loss of water weight, which occurs when the body sweats to cool down working muscles.

That quick drop in "weight" on the scale has little to do with a reduction of stored fat.[1] As soon as you hydrate from the substantial amount of water lost, you will have gained back all of the weight dropped. A loss that is more than 1 or 2 pounds at most might be a sign that you are losing muscular tissue and I am not just speaking in regards to skeletal muscle, but vital organ tissue as well. So you now see how dangerous those fad diets that claim a loss of 10 pounds or more in a week really are!)

One last trick that can assist your fat loss efforts, as well as your muscle building efforts, is to consume foods that are closer to their natural state. I want to make clear at this point in time that I am not telling you to shop at a "health food" store in search of "organic" and "natural" produce. Your typical grocery store, such as Wal-Mart, supplies a plentiful array of fruits, vegetables and other foodstuffs that are far better than what are sold at supposed "health food" stores...since the only difference in their respective inventory is the prices—there is *absolutely no benefit over shopping at a health food store over a general grocery store.*

Now, when choosing your food selection for your both your fat loss and optimal muscle building diet (which are essentially the same thing, save for caloric differences) select foods that are closer to nature, such as fresh fruit and vegetables; breads, oats and brand products; lean meats and low fat dairy products. A heavy consumption of processed sugars can have a negative affect on your insulin levels, thus hindering your fat loss efforts due to an oversaturation of your muscles' glycogen stores resulting in more circulating blood glucose being shuttled toward fat storage. Excessive insulin levels due to heavy refined sugar consumption also negatively affect your muscle growth, as anabolic hormones, particularly growth hormone and testosterone, are obstructed by high levels of insulin.

When consuming a diet of foodstuffs that are closer to their natural form, your body actually requires energy to digest them and make them utilizable—as opposed to refine sugars that are readily available to enter your blood stream—so you are actually burning calories in the process of trying to use the calories contained in these foods. So all and all, consuming a diet full of foods closer to their natural states not only provides a greater quantity of satisfying bulk with fewer calories than most processed foods and supplies innumerable compounds that positively affect your health and your muscle gaining/fat loss efforts, but also burns calories merely in their digestion. As for refined sugars in your dietary equation, you do not have to eliminate them; they may even be incredibly beneficial at times of lethargy and ill focus… just try to keep them to a minimum.

What About Supplements?

Taking advantage of the fact that most people are naturally lazy, quite a number of other people with little, if any, interest in anything except money—and with no regard for the truth—have devoted many years of their time and hundreds of millions of dollars to brainwash the general public on the subject of nutrition and muscle growth….I am referring to the people who should know better…and frequently do know better. People whom, while claiming to be the strongest supporters of the field of health and fitness are in fact its worst enemies: the supplement/bodybuilding and health food industries.

Bodybuilders need to be more intelligent when it comes to pursuing their interests and more economically efficient with investing only in things that further their ability instead of causing harm…in addition to not break their wallet. There was a time when bodybuilders (non-steroid users at the time), powerlifters (though at the time they were called "odd" lifters), Olympic weightlifters (back then they actually lifted the weights and were penalized for throwing the weight on the clean or any jerking on the press) and strongmen, though many years ago, ate only a balanced or even semi-balanced diet and consumed no protein, creatine or other supposed "muscle building" supplements of any kind.

Individual such as Steve Reeves, Tommy Kono, Bob Peoples, Pudgy Stockton, Louis Cyr and John Grimek did not have access to the immense variety of ominously concocted nutritional and muscle building/fat loss supplements presented in the magazines today…and yet, all of these individuals were able to building stunningly powerful and muscular physiques—the likes of which are rare to see even today. But as most of the professional bodybuilders today do not take the time nor the effort to dispel the fallacies of "magic muscle building elixirs" and anti-fat powders or pills, etc.—most choose to do just the opposite by recommending neophytic bodybuilders to spend hundreds of dollars a month on these worthless products—, thus it is up to you, the consumer, to do your research.

The consumer is the individual who chooses to purchase their product; they are not forced to buy the products by the manufacturer…at least not in a free market. It is the responsibility of the consumer to do their homework when it comes to investing in something; whether it is a home, a family, a business or their body. Consequently, the consumers of the supplement industry are, more often than not, the misguided individuals that believe that we need to consume additional quantities of nutrients by way of supplementation, as apparently the diet of a bodybuilder—supposedly a high protein diet— does not supply the needed quantities that we need and that these extra *supplemental* nutrients will allow us to attain the greatest rate of growth possible.

Firstly, as for the needing of supplemented nutrients because of a poor diet, even if this were true, chronic poor foods choices, even with supplements, would leave you deficient in the thousands of plant compounds (polyphenols and phytochemicals) essential to good health.[2] The word supplement means precisely that: to supplement the diet. The mystical claims of ultimate health and of building muscle through a diet are erroneous. There is no such thing as an ultimate state of health, only an optimum—your optimum—state of health, dictated by your genetics, and there is not a single supplement on earth, and I repeat, not a single one that *produces* muscle growth. Some will defend with, "Well, what if we are not getting enough nutrients in our food…what if we actually need more than is suggested in order to gain the most muscle possible?"

The fact is that when it comes to the vitamins and minerals, we need little in the way of these micronutrients as they, as the prefix *micro* implies, are needed in small amounts—demonstrated particularly with vitamin B12. The human body conserves vitamin B-12 very efficiently, as Dr. Victor Herbert, MD, JD, an expert in folic acid and B-12 metabolism, wrote in *Modern Nutrition in Health and Disease*, "This almost total conservation of vitamin B-12 explains why pure vegetarians who eat almost no vitamin B-12 takes decades to develop deficiency of the vitamin." The average B-12 stores in humans range from 2 to 5 mg, and "there is little evidence for significant catabolism, of vitamin B-12, by man, and it is probable that loss occurs only by excretion, mainly in bile."[3]

Vitamin C has had the greatest publicity in the public, from its supposed magical cold prevention and curing capabilities due to its antioxidant capabilities. However, researchers have found that the vitamin C in apples is responsible for only a small portion of the antioxidant activity. Instead, almost all of this activity in apples is from polyphenols. Indeed, previous studies have shown that a 500-milligram vitamin C pill might

act as a pro-oxidant.[4] Oxidative activity is catabolic; it is
the breakdown of tissue and that is where you can harm
someone. What is actually needed in vitamin C, and is
recommended by all reputable nutritionists, is *only* 75
mg a day; that is provided in one orange or a glass of
most fruit juices. Anymore than 75 mg a day will not
force your body to utilize, to any further extent, anymore
than 75 mg…and trying to force hundreds or thousands
of mgs of vitamin C down your throat will only cause far
more harm than good.

If you want to know what the body's biological
requirements are, consult an RDI reference. But
even to this, some people will declare that the RDI's
recommendations are only nutritional minimums.
However, the truth is that the RDI's recommendations
are *generous* margins, allowing almost double than the
actual needed amount in some cases.

Another defense for supplements some will use is that
because of over-farming, the soil has become depleted
and lacks the essential vitamins and minerals needed to
sustain us. These people, however, lack the understanding
that humans are not the only life on earth that requires
nutrients in order to grow. If the soil were as depleted as
many people claim then none of our produce would look
as they did 100 or even 50 years ago. And since I have
yet to hear an old man yelling in a senile rage that those
apples don't look as they use too, I have little doubt that
they are.

With the industrial enriching of the soil, pesticides
and preservatives, we have the opportunity to enjoy
produce from all over the world from are own separate
corners of the globe. Never has man been able to enjoy

the sweet fruits and rich vegetables from many different cultures at any whim—all the result of the advanced industrialization of farming.

* * *

Being fanatical on maximizing muscle growth, bodybuilders of all degrees of bewilderment convene, intellectually, on the bromide of emphasizing tremendous amounts of extra protein, purporting its necessity for the growth and repair a bodybuilder's muscles. However, contrary to what most of the public thinks—believing that protein requirements varying by activity (e.g. muscle building, dieting, increasing strength, etc.)—, protein requirements are *not* contingent on activity, but on bodyweight.

Unobstructed by ineffable notions discharged from the muscle/fitness magazines, we understand that because muscle is not mostly comprised of protein, but of water, we circumvent this propagated protein fallacy and understand that carbohydrates, as the suffix hydrate implies, hydrates the muscle as a result of holding three times its weight in water within the muscle.

The argument that building big muscles requires a large amount of protein is based on an idea that you will build 5 pounds of *dry* muscular tissue (without any water in it, which is quite substantial when you think of muscle being 72 percent water) in a week's time, every week. This is the naive neophytic faith in the professional bodybuilders' quixotic testament that can be summed up in the statement "If I train long enough and consume a lot of protein I will inevitably produce a mountain of muscle." This belief is so powerful among neophyte bodybuilders that an advertisement that ran through the 60's and well into the 70's in a popular muscle magazine stated that if you drank their "special" formula you would gain one pound of muscle a day—this drink consisted of a cheap protein powder with a gallon or more of whole milk. The results? ...well let's just say that it was a very profitable time for tailors who had plenty of work letting out pants and shirts for consistently growing fatter and fatter customers, who then came back in six months to have their cloths returned to their original size after losing all of that gained body fat.

In all reality, stimulating one pound of muscle tissue a week is a phenomenal achievement. And since there are only 600 calories in a pound of muscle, if a bodybuilder were to stimulate a pound of muscle growth over a week's time, he would need to consume an extra 14 grams of protein, equaling an extra 86 calories each day. This, although, is only accomplished with individuals performing a workout in an intensity fashion to *stimulate* growth, not by his food consumption. The truth of muscular growth is that the nutrition aspect of it is only *secondary*, as research with animals has shown that muscular growth can occur on a zero calorie diet, constituted of just water, if they were exercised properly beforehand.[5]

In closing for this rhetoric on supplementation, I would like to say that I only support the intelligent use of two supplements, outside a personal physician's instructions. During menstruation women can lose a great quantity of the mineral iron. This can cause chronic fatigue, irritability, weakness and brittle nails among other things. Therefore, for women who do not consume very iron rich foodstuffs I do recommend a low-grade iron supplement. The last supplement that I recommend, or rather, that I would not protest, is a simple multivitamin for bodybuilders dieting for a contest when they are at the point where they are taking in only 1500 or less' calories a day.

Part VI
Life or Death

"Nothing discernable to the eye of the spirit is more brilliant or obscure than man; nothing is more formidable, complex, mysterious, and infinite. There is a prospect greater than the sea, and it is the sky; there is a prospect greater than the sky, and it is the human soul."

Victor Hugo,
"Les Miserables"

"An individual's self-esteem stems from a sense of control over reality. Whenever we carry out a conscious effort, such as, completing a record Bench Press, an A+ in school or writing a book, we feel a specific power rising, a sense of will. The abundant self-esteem associated with successful people flows from their having achieved goals by exerting the proper effort - long range. People are not successful due to an accident of birth; they took the time and expended the necessary effort to develop their self-respect. They sufficiently value life and happiness to exert complete effort. As a result, they experience what Aristotle referred to as the "crown of all virtues": Pride."

Mike Mentzer

"The victory of success is half won when one gains the habit of setting goals and achieving them. Even the most tedious chore will become endurable as you parade through each day convinced that every task, no matter how menial or boring, brings you closer to fulfilling your dreams."

Og Mandino

10

The Role of Values

Bodybuilding is truly a virtuous act of a man qua life. It is virtuous for the reason that bodybuilding is one of the most *selfish* things that one can perform. When choosing the commendable endeavor of bodybuilding one, implicitly or consciously, recognizes their *own* self-worth and the importance of *their* happiness. Bodybuilding is done for the betterment of oneself. It involves two of the most personal and selfishly intimate acts man can perform, and possesses the one fundament individual right that makes possible all other human rights: the right to property, i.e., the right to the product of one's own efforts and the choice of its use.

Bodybuilding requires goal-oriented thought (intensely personal and intimate) and it is founded upon the pursuit of one's own happiness—whether it is muscular prowess or sexual attractiveness to one's preferred sex or the arousing pride one obtains from actualizing their potential with their own effort and passionate desire to achieve a dream....To understand the meaning and vital human necessity of goal-oriented pursuit one must first understand the role of values.

The Role of Values

A value, as Ayn Rand precisely defined, is something that one acts to gain and keep; a virtue, Ayn Rand further contended, is the action one performs to gain and keep it. But a value is not a primary; a value presupposes an answer to the question: a value to whom and for what?

All values rest upon an essential primary, i.e. a principle standard (a fundamental value). Man judges the worth of his values in accord to his fundamental value, thus, his values exist in a hierarchy of importance—rated by the degree that they are consonant with or insignificant or inimical to his principle standard. However, value presupposes a purpose and the requirement of action in the face of an alternative. And since man is man, being a living organism, and since the fundamental value of an organism is itself, i.e. its own life, man's nature dictates that man qua man's survival requires that he upholds his life and the maintenance of it as the ultimate standard of value.

Yet man is a being of a volitional consciousness and he must choose his ethical standard from an array of conflicting philosophies that he is confronted with from the cradle—predominantly by an atavistic, tyrannical catechism of faith based sacrificial standards from which man today, and has long been, attacked with.

What moral standard an individual chooses, explicitly and consciously through study and deliberation or arbitrarily by his subconscious and cultural consensus, afflicts his value assessment of all things he encounters. One's principle ethical conviction dictates how they assess all values, such as, bodybuilding, whether they see it as (a) a virtuous act of presenting oneself as man the hero, capable of achieving goals and gaining self-esteem, (b) an immoral evil of "selfishness", or (c) an amoral activity that is not worth contemplating; love, whether they see love as (a) a selfish, intimate admiration of another individual's virtues, not vices, that are in concert with one's own idolized values…gaining emotional pleasure in their presence—knowing the importance of oneself and their worthiness of love by the acknowledgement of their virtues, (b) as an "unconditional" duty to thy mother, thy father and thy neighbor…being outside one's "self" qua moral choice, or (c) an illusory term that exists only in romantic novels, having nothing to do with reality; and such issues as sex, whether they view sex as (a) one of the most important aspects of man's life that is not to be addressed with promiscuous abandon nor approached unconscientiously or indifferently, (b) as an evil that is beyond immoral and an outright act of moral degradation, or (c) as a evil that is "instinctive" to man and thus unavoidable, so believing that it should be performed in an animalistic orgy with no moral concern or personal value of the other individual.

A rationally selfish man, a being of true self-esteem, acknowledges that his life is his highest moral value from which all his values follow, an individual who assesses all of the previous value-issues with the first premise.

Now understand when I speak of being selfish I do not speak of an individual who sacrifices others to himself, but of an individual who truly understands the importance of the "self." Selfish literally means *concern with one's own interests.* Someone who sacrifices others to himself is not selfish—to be selfish is to be an individualist. He is but a parasite, a selfless individual. Just as those who sacrifice themselves to others, he lives second-hand—off of the effort and/or approval of others (whether he is a manipulator of the altruistic and confused or the fodder to some benefactor—both are parasites: one of the material goods of others, one of the spiritual consent of others). To be "selfless" is not to be pro-man, but anti-man—man is a being, by his nature, of the ego.

In order for man to be *selfless* he must renounce himself, immolate, and abrogate the self to the needs, wants, desires, and demands of others. To see the anti-man nature of selflessness we recognize that one cannot be born selfless nor can one live being truly selfless, it is contradictory to man's nature. Sacrifice is only possible to those who have come to selfishly value something and choose to part with it for a lesser or non-value—it is not a sacrifice is you do not care for something personally. Those who are truly selfish realize that the primordial sacrificial altar of the self, rooted deep in the nature of altruism is the worst form of immorality that has allowed such unspeakable atrocities in history—such as communist Russia and Nazi Germany—to take place under the title of the moral, the good, the just.

In order to be selfish one must first understand that *his* life is *his* highest value, and because of which, his ultimate standard is life, not servitude—to live for his own selfish interest. To be selfish is to stand on *your* own reason with *plerophory*, not on faith nor the vote of some disembodied pragmatic consensus called the public interest, and take responsibility for your own actions, judgment, thoughts and feelings—as such things are all functions of the *self*; functions that are impossible to a truly selfless person.

In standing for your self-interest you are obligated by the law of identity to respect the *rights* of others, if you wish your own rights to be recognized and respected. To assert that it is in one's selfish interest to rob a bank or steal a Porsche is an utterly irrational dropping of context and a complete conscious evasion of the law of causality. You have two outcomes of such an action: (a) you are caught immediately and are imprisoned with various shady inimical characters or (b) you are in a perpetual state of fear and neurotic anticipation of every siren, every news report being the police on your heels…. Now to whom would that be considered in their self-interest? In order to achieve goals and values of your own self-interest you are obligated by the law of causality to be rational.

Selfishness presupposes a purpose: the maintenance and betterment of one's own life. To do so man must hold three things as supreme and ruling values of his life: reason, purpose and self-esteem. To be selfish is to be conscious of the enormous responsibility of *living one's own life*—which means, the pursuit and attainment of values. For a much more comprehensive and dramatic elucidation of why it is right and moral for man to be selfish I advise that you read Ayn Rand's novel, *The Fountainhead.*

* * *

Now it is important to understand that the recognition of the worth of a value to you conditions the emotional response and conscious degree of motivation to gain and/ or keep it.

Periodically, all bodybuilders have times where lethargy and ill focus accompany them into the gym and they lack the intrepid motivation necessary for a hardcore, Heavy Duty workout. Reasons for such, varying from emotional indolence to merely felling out of sorts, can vary from conflicts with a loved one, anxiety from work or loss of an important value. However, what I have found to be the main proprietor of motivational abasement for bodybuilders is the loss of focus or a diminishing understanding of a value's importance to themselves. No, this is not a sign of moral weakness or a psychological defect; it only means that you do not full grasp the vital importance of that value to you. I have had periods where I drudged through a workout, finishing with only a sense of a half-ass effort and disappointment—consequently accompanied by meager progress. It was not until I comprehensively reflected on and assessed my prior emotional behavior and thoughts of my training that I was able to indicate a percolating error in my value assessment of building a more powerful and muscular physique.

I was losing sight of the purpose of my training and the necessity of a hardcore, intense psyche required to attain my goal. I have found, time and again, that writing stokes the passionate, purposeful fire at the base of my motivation, fueling me to push through the muscular agony and emotional torment inexorable in Heavy Duty high intensity training, onward to greater growth. As the result of a full understanding of the value of greater muscular size and strength to my very important goal, I gained approximately five pounds of muscle in slightly under a month.

I suggest that if you find that you are having regular spells of lethargy and have made sure that you are training correctly—avoiding overtraining that can cause lingering emotional and physical exhaustion—write down the importance of your efforts in the gym...why it is vital to your happiness and self-esteem. Write paragraphs or even pages about why the achievement of a greater, more muscular and powerful body is crucial to you. Write about things that inspire you and things that stimulate an electrical shudder down your spine in emotional excitement. Read philosophical books or romantic/ heroic novels of man pitted against the odds, only to beat all probability and end victorious, or study motivational pictures and paintings that personally signify heroic effort and true motivation. When you are in periods of passionate ambition and relentless motivation write down and attempt to describe such exaltation for future reference.

Keep at ready these instruments of effervescent tinder, for when you feel insipid and your passionate fire is in a motivational flounder; reflect upon your writings and favorite passages from inspirational works. Remember that *nothing of value comes to man automatically—even motivation.* If you want to achieve your goals you must make the unrelenting effort to reaffirm a value's imperative meaning to your standard of life. But do not take these obstacles halfheartedly, they are your battles to bear and, if you win, they will leave you with the scars of triumph forever engraved in your being...or in the tenor of Maxwell Maltz, "We find no real satisfaction or happiness in life without obstacles to conquer and goals to achieve."

11

The Workout: A Reason to Fight!

*"If you greatly desire something, have the
guts to stake everything on obtaining it."*
Brendan Francis

As one walks upon the earth for which the iron beasts
dwell, a person of intellectual uncertainty, bound by the
captive indolence of an ill motivation, begins to wonder
and then ask of themselves, "What will become of me?
…How does one enter the grounds for which there is
no alternative to acquiring one's goal than a physical and
emotional seriousness wholly coveted, yet relished only
by those who take seemingly unbearable struggles head-
on with no second thought as to the difficulty?"

Know dear reader that this can *only* be done by
understanding the utter personal *necessity* of surmounting
the enemy, a negative, a loss of that which gives you
everything you live for. By entering the gym with a
declaration of war!—viewing your workouts with
intellectual and moral certainty and righteousness.
Knowing that the stratagem of your victory is perfect and
the only further need to obtain your goal is to execute the
attack with every ounce of your being put forth…with
necessity of this effort fueled by the acknowledgement

of the importance of a value to your moral-psychological wellbeing.

This is the psyche that one needs in order to proliferate the intensity needed to stimulate *life*. Yes life, as life is an ever-active and ever-progressive state; for without progression and growth comes death.

The state of mind needed to be worthy of progress must be one of a hero about to enter battle—purpose and passion overwhelm all the senses of your body; perspiring an energy that creates trepidation in the air around you, resulting in anyone who comes close to you without such a state of being becoming tortured by the intensity of your desire. But now comes forth the question of how does one come to such a height? How does one go about cultivating such a state of impervious, purposeful focus?

Realize that this is a state of mind that one is not born with nor happens to come upon by chance. This is a focus that was cultivated by a purpose and the necessity of obtaining a value. Characterized by the obsessive temperament of relentlessly striving for more, better, the greatest that one is possible of. The individuals of this nature are distinctive from the orthodox, distinct as being truly motivated—once this stratum of individuals enter the grounds of the gym or their chosen exigent field of trial, their mind fosters an imperturbable passionate focus towards the pursuit of moving mountains and lifting the heavens themselves!

Now this mindset is not an easy one to achieve, as it requires an unbridled acknowledgement of a value's meaning to oneself. A psyche that is not simply cultured in a sheer discharge of an in-the-moment passionate urge. To develop the needed mindset to undergo what would be accurately described as an effort of fighting for your life, you need an undeniable, irreplaceable value to pursue. The human body has developed as such an efficient survival organism that it has evolutionarily fashioned psychological barriers in order to avoid devouring all of its energy needed in order to flee from life threatening situations. It is only the utter need to acquire or protect a value that will allow you to be able to tap into your full human potential, to tap into 100 percent of your possible intensity. Every human being possesses the potential of expressing 100 percent of their possible strength at any given moment…but such a potential is sealed deep in the depths of your mind, restrained by psychological defensive barriers that percolate interceptive negative thoughts and emotions that intensify once you tread upon subsequent rung after subsequent rung of the intensifying layers.

There is an unignorable tendency to want to give up when the intensity really starts to build—especially on the more demanding exercises as the deadlift and the squat. Nevertheless, remember that yours is a voluntary consciousness; you possess the latent human strength and *will* to bite the bullet and achieve personal goals. The attempt to devote 100 percent of one's energies into one action would be best valuably compared to running in front of a Mac truck (symbolizing true high intensity training: a virtue) in exchange for saving the life of one you hold so dear (muscle growth: a value).

The action of a truly high intensity workout demands mental and physical courage. Nothing less than an irrefutable need to fight on and stake your precious energy on the pursuit of a value will allow you to push beyond your previous limits. The higher the level of intensity you reach, for which you come closer to 100 percent of your *momentary* muscular ability, the easier it becomes to get back up to that same level. But remember, one needs to strive for better and higher grounds of success. Mike Mentzer best described the bodybuilder as a progressionist not a perfectionist...for without progression life becomes stagnant and dies. To the bodybuilder, perfection is merely a stepping-stone to greater heights of possibility.

*   *   *

Using passionately stirring and epically triumphant classical music such as Tchaikovsky, Richard Strauss or Frederick Chopin and the heavy driving music of hard rock or heavy metal before and during a workout has helped me in cultivating vivid imagery of epically powerful struggles and, ultimately, victory. I have found that music that epitomizes man as a hero, up against seemingly insurmountable, teratological odds...struggling through a heroic battle that requires every ounce of passion, energy and emotional release for what he is fighting for that ultimately ends in victory for the hero, intensifies my focus and my emotional seriousness.

Using visions of life threatening situations as well can help you to draw upon higher levels of strength during your workout. For example, while doing underhand pulldowns or chins, visualize that you are hanging off the edge of a cliff—do you continue holding on and pull yourself back up to the ledge for life or let go and succumbing to oblivion. Or while performing a squat or bench-pressing movement, seeing that the weight bearing down upon you is an immense object that is attempting to douse the flame of yours and a loved one's life.

(This is what a hero is: one who fights for and stakes everything on *their* values, goals and dreams. Heroics are of the utmost need of man today in our morally bankrupt, self-sacrificing despondent culture. Every valiant man dreams of the glory of an epic battle, fighting selfishly—whether they implicitly know it or not—for their values, their morals, their love; the kind of battle that penetrates the waters of history and echoes with whispers of the tales of such astronomical struggles and triumphs of the mind and of the body. Stories perpetuating such events began coming forth in the stories of ancient Greek mythology, of mighty gods and men in the throws of earthly climatic combat and war against unearthly monsters; upon which cultures were changed and legends were born.)

Man, as a Hero

"Of the many ideals which in youth gave life a meaning and radiance missing from the chilly perspectives of middle age, one at least has remained with me as bright and satisfying as ever before—the shameless worship of heroes. In an age that would level everything and reverence nothing, I take my stand with Victorian Carlyle, and light my candles, like Mirandola before Plato's shrines of great men....For why should we stand reverent before waterfalls and mountain tops, or a summer moon on a quiet sea, and not before the highest miracle of all—a man who is both great and good?
Will Durant, philosopher and historian

In *The Romantic Manifesto*, Ayn Rand presents two cultural manifestations of man that have been the full embodiment of the two distinct alternatives of the philosophical view of life for man. "Consider two statues of man: one as a Greek god, the other as a deformed medieval monstrosity. Both are metaphysical estimates of man; both are projections of the artist's view of man's nature; both are concretized representations of the philosophy of their respective cultures."

In this comparison we are dealing with two cultures of man's philosophical extremes: the ancient Greek and the medievalist. One culture chose to represent man qua man as they believed and knew him to be possible of achieving, the other chose to represent man as something that they did not have to look up to nor strive to achieve. One chose to worship *man's* limitless and magnanimous potential, one chose to disregard man as possible of achieving beyond the feeling and urges of the moment. One loved *man* as being capable of achieving his values and of being a hero, one despised man for his capability of achieving and of being a hero. One loved life; one only feared death and thus resented life. Conflicting between these two philosophies are their respective *ethical standard*, that ultimate value which they refer to in order to evaluate values and, therefore, virtues.

...In what way do you envision life, better yet, how do you believe life should be lived? The effort you put forth in the gymnasium, and in all goal-oriented (value seeking) endeavors in your life, is a metaphysical re-creation of how you view life and how you believe it should be lived—it is an art form. Art being a selective re-creation of reality according to an artist's metaphysical value judgments—that is, according to what the artist believes to be ultimately true and important about the nature of reality and man.

If one holds the ideals of life by the noble ethos of the ancient Greek, the deepest depths of passion one has for life will be expressed through a relentless passion that drives their spirit to ever-greater heights of exaltation and triumph.

The ancient Greek choose to reject the mystic cats, dogs and cow-headed monstrosities enshrined and worshiped by the Egyptians; conceiving their gods as perfect human beings embodying all of the beautiful and noble virtues that man is capable of. The ancient Greek chose to taste the forbidden fruit of knowledge, to covet the fire of the gods...refusing the alternative of being obedient to some unknowable zero, to being incapable of understanding—they chose to be man rather than non-man.

Ancient Greece was the birth place of reason and of the first love of man, specifically, the first acknowledgement of his rights; that ultimately lead to the founding fathers full recognition of man's individual rights: that man's life is his and the good is for him to live it.

Individuals who hold their morals by the standards first conceived by the ancient Greek know that their efforts are neither in vain of some spiritually omnipotent entity, nor a culturally accepted duty of mediocrity, but a statement that this is a selfish act for their happiness and coincides with their pleasures, joys, desires and dreams. That their intense physically and intellectually demanding struggles for self-improvement are an expression of their love of life and how they know life as a man of reason should live it: fighting for their values and never letting anything hold them back from obtaining it, even if it means their life! They fight, romantically and heroically, for what man could be and ought to be.

This is the attitude one has if they see their life as an unprecedented joy; that every activity—intellectual or physical—is meant for them, for their happiness. That pursuing and achieving a value by the reliance of man's power to think awards man with the emotional and conceptual manifestation and recognition of the sum of all virtues: *pride.* Thus, allowing him to gain the greatest happiness that man can experience that is of vital necessity to a man who desires to live on earth: *self-esteem,* that is to say, the knowledge and certainty that his mind is competent to think and he is worthy of happiness… worthy of living.

Then again, if one upholds the pathos ethoses of the medieval era we can readily observe their philistine sort in the slums and malignant hovels of despair along with the conceding minds of the ritual majority. The men of the depressed occult have no desire to go on and to live out their former ideals, surrendering to the depraved impression that one cannot be both ideal and moral in life, they compromise all of their values to try and be practical by the standard of our intellectuals, down to the level of stagnation and moral rot.

Their view of how man should be is not the glorious hero that has the capacity for the most remarkable acts: heroically pursuing his own values and his happiness with moral righteousness! No, theirs is a view of how man should be that is corrupted by their vision of what they allow themselves to observe what man is by the standards of the those who tergiversate reality, reason and justice— the intellectual cowards and the frauds of the mind…the looters, the rapists, racists, pedophiles and murders of the world. They crouch in a wallow of moral despondency, having the depressive conviction of, "Why dream of such heroic individuals when they can never exist in reality?" These are the people who, if ever, pursuing a job, gymnastic and aesthetic scholastics, a relationship, or what have you, dismissingly do the bare minimum or lesser of the activity. Doing so only for the simple and sole goal of performing their "*social duty*," so they can return to their hole of anguish and let the moments of their life lapse by.

These are the two ultimate alternatives of every man, woman and child: to let their life err into rot and stoop to the level of an intellectual stillborn…or to go for the gusto, take the bull by the horns and just grab life by the balls and take its for all its worth and be a hero.

Understand that a hero *is not* some supernatural being or abnormality in the history of mankind; a hero is not born from the womb; a hero is not an impossible ideal in reality. What a hero is in reality *is* a status only achievable by man, by a volitional choice; a hero comes about only by a *choice* to fight for one's values, their desired standard of life—a facility *every* individual possesses; a hero *is* an individual who recognizes that only in being rational are they capable of living and of achieving the ideal, that ideals are practical if based on rational premises. A hero is one who understands the role of values and the unprecedented value of their own life. Therefore, they understand the value of the life of every individual and, on moral grounds, respects them with same respect he gives everything in reality—rationality. A hero, a rational individual, is the *only* being capable of truly loving another individual and of selfishly fighting for the one who they love, whether it is a friend, their child or a lover. A hero possesses, what Aristotle called, the crown of all virtues: the stature of a *Magnanimous Being*.

*   *   *

A bodybuilder is one who understands the heroics that man is capable of and emboldens this strong and virtuous stature with the actualization of their body's full muscular potential and their mind's continuous conceptual growth. Just as the ancient Greek fashioned man as a hero, epitomizing him as a god, from rich and pure marble as his medium and a chisel and a mallet as his tools, so too does a bodybuilder fashion his body as a hero. Except, instead of marble as his medium and a chisel and mallet as his tools, a bodybuilder uses his body as his medium and his tools are that which the ancient Greek strived to embody in their sculptures: intellectual sweat, a relentless effort for striving for one's individual perfection, the potential muscular beauty man's body is capable of, and the courage to preserver through the throws of struggle and intense effort....

If you decide to take on your life's goals, including that of a more muscular body, with a defeatist philosophy and philistine attitude you will never obtain your esteemed values. Do not look upon the ventures of life as ordeals of ever-imminent stress, anxiety, pain and ultimately defeat. Take pride in the difficult of your tasks ahead and the fact that you are capable of failing. Use that possibility of failure and losing that what is precious to you as fuel to motivate yourself to give it ***everything*** you have...deep down to that last drop of energy, deep in the well of your very being. Embolden in your struggle the emotional release of pride, knowing that this effort only stands to bring you one-step closer to actualizing your goal!

You must focus on *every* repetition as a set of itself—important, vital to your growth—bestowing the same impenetrable concentration as that last repetition requires. As your task becomes more demanding, rep by rep, second by second, moment by moment, you must hold firmly in your mind why…why this pain, this agony is necessary and important to you! Mentally repeat to yourself your goal and how every ounce of pain of every succeeding repetition only deepens your focus; every second of agony only strengthens your resolve. Don't just be a bodybuilder…be a hero.

Of Mind & Body

"And yet it moves!"

Galileo Galilei

Throughout this book you have been inundated with a broad spectrum of topics extending from physiology to philosophy to nutrition. Nevertheless, the abroad that has been laid down was required for one purpose. This book is ultimately a general and rudimentary means of discovering the objective truth of man's body. As I will reiterate, reality is the ultimate arbiter of truth. It is a conceptual adherence to reality that is the deciding factor in your efforts of attaining a greater body—intellectually and physically.

Life as a rational being is utterly enthralling with all of its potentialities. And it is our faculty of reason, as the rational being, that allows man us pursue our values and attain our long-range goals in the most efficacious manner possible—through logic. With logic as our method of goal-oriented pursuit, we are capable of achieving what is only possible to man: gaining and keeping his values—obtaining true, noncontradictory joy. What can possibly be more exhilarating and literally breathtaking than striving for what man could be and ought to be, and achieving that!

303

When studying the science of bodybuilding through the means of logic you begin to learn about the nature of the human mind…about thought itself. Through intensive and passionate study of the proper, logical manner in which to conduct your bodybuilding efforts, you soon become splendidly aware of a residing desire to facilitate an ever-growing hunger for expanding your awareness; that is only capable of being satisfied by extending your knowledge to other avenues of study and of fervescent passion. Such things as, discovering all of the intricacies of the human body within neuroanatomy, cardiology, osteology or anything else within the realm of human physiology; learning of the full potential of the human mind through an undertaking of the study of philosophy; studying the architectural magnificence of modern skyscrapers that break-free of nephological bounds; or maybe even discovering the nature of romantic love with finding an individual who sets ablaze a passionate romantic love between the two of you.

It is a man of true integrity and of moral guidance who does not insult even a moment of his precious life by not pursuing greater knowledge and strength. Do not allow your intense flames of aspiring towards achieving your dreams dwindle from the mediocrity and uncertainty of those of a weak willed ilk. Do not believe that your noble ideals, your values, your goals, and your happiness are not practical or worth fighting for. Let your muscles be an expression of you, consecrating your life from this moment on towards pursuing your life qua your goals, your passions, your values, your dreams; your liberty from those who would only try to diminish your self-esteem; and, ultimately, towards the pursuit of your happiness— strive to be a true bodybuilder, of mind and body.

References:

A Reasoned Approach to Exercise

[1]–Lange, *Uber Funktionelle Anpassung* USW, Berlin, Julius Springer, 1917.

[2]–Steinhaus, Arthur. *Towards an Understanding of Health and Physical Education*. WM. C. Brown Company Publishers. P, 134, 1963

Individual Potential

[1,6,9]–Little J. *Max Contraction Training*. Chicago: Library of Congress Cataloguing in Publication Data. P, 32,33,49,57. 2003

[2,4,7]–Mentzer M. and Little J. *High-Intensity Training the Mike Mentzer Way*. Contemporary Books, Chicago. P, 14, 15, 17, 74. 2003

[3,5,8,10]–McGuff D. *Ultimate Exercise Bulletin Number 1*. Chicago: Library of Congress Cataloguing in Publication Data. 1997

Supplementary Concerns

[1, 3]–Lightsey, David. *Muscles, Speed & Lies*. The Globe Pequot Press., 2006.

[2, 5]–Darden, Ellington. *The Nautilus Nutrition Book*. Chicago: Contemporary Books, Inc., P. 278. 1981

ALEX FEE is an individual who fell in love with the heroic image of the bodybuilder at a very young age. Along the way in his years of training and study he met a man named John Little, who completely changed his life. After a period of tutelage under John Little and the works of the late Mike Mentzer and Arthur Jones, Alex became captivated by the philosophy of Ayn Rand and found himself inculcated with a tsunami of logic and rationality that set the cornerstone in his intellectual foundation.